Mr A.R.I. Al-Sheikhli
Friday, 22nd August, 1997

GW00703376

EPONYMISTS IN MEDICINE

Sir James Paget
The Rise of Clinical Surgery

Shirley Roberts

Editor-in-Chief: Hugh L'Etang

Royal Society of Medicine Services Limited

Royal Society of Medicine Services Limited
1 Wimpole Street London W1M 8AE
7 East 60th Street New York NY 10022

British Library Cataloguing in Publication Data

Roberts, S.
  James Paget.
  1. Medicine. Paget, James
  I. Title II. Series
  610' .92' 4
  ISBN 0-905958-99-3

Editorial and production services by Diane Crofter-Harris, Devizes, Wiltshire

Design and typesetting by Mehmet Hussein/Medilink Design

Printed in Great Britain by Henry Ling Ltd, at the Dorset Press, Dorchester

Acknowledgements

Many people responded generously to my appeals for information and advice as I worked on this project. Lieutenant-Colonel Sir Julian Paget, Bart, great-grandson of Sir James, made available the unpublished family history 'The Pagets of Great Yarmouth', with its numerous illustrations, and provided much additional information from his personal knowledge. Without his help the task could not have been accomplished.

Several of my colleagues at Prince Henry's Hospital, Melbourne—Dr Leila Cavanagh, Mr Alistair Davidson, and Dr Graeme McKinnon—helped me with information on aspects of pathology and microbiology. Dr Peter Verco of Adelaide kindly gave me permission to quote from his book *Millers, Masons, and Medicine*.

In England I visited the British Library and the libraries of the Royal Society of Medicine, the Royal College of Surgeons, the Wellcome Institute for the History of Medicine, and the City of Norwich. I am grateful for the expert assistance I received at all these institutions. Miss Janet Foster and Mr Geoffrey Yeo, Archivists of St Bartholomew's Hospital, answered my queries and directed me to additional sources of information.

In Melbourne I received valuable assistance from the librarians of the Royal Australasian College of Surgeons, the University of Melbourne, the State Reference Library, Prince Henry's Hospital, and the Australian Medical Association.

I am indebted to Professor AGL Shaw and to Professor Harold Attwood, both of whom read the manuscript and gave me the benefit of their knowledge and experience.

Illustrations

Notable Events

1793 Death of John Hunter
1797 Battle of Camperdown
1798 Battle of the Nile
      Edward Jenner introduces vaccination against smallpox
1799 Marriage of Samuel Paget and Sarah Tolver
1814 Birth of James Paget
1830 James Paget begins surgical apprenticeship
1832 Britain suffers its first cholera epidemic
1834 James Paget becomes a student at St Bartholomew's
      Hospital
1835 James Paget and Richard Owen discover the Trichina
      parasite
1836 Paget admitted to Membership of the Royal College of
      Surgeons
      Paget becomes engaged to Lydia North
1838 Paget nearly dies of typhus
1842 Paget begins work on the pathology catalogue of the
      Hunterian Museum of the Royal College of Surgeons
1843 Paget becomes the first Warden of the College at
      St Bartholomew's Hospital
      Death of Mrs Paget, James's mother
1844 Marriage of James Paget and Lydia North
1847 Paget is elected Arris and Gale Professor at the Royal
      College of Surgeons and appointed assistant surgeon at
      the Hospital
      James Young Simpson reads his historic paper on ether as
      an anaesthetic agent
1849 Paget completes the pathology catalogue of the Hunterian
      Museum
      The second cholera epidemic occurs and John Snow begins
      his important work on the spread of the disease
1850 Elizabeth Blackwell visits St Bartholomew's Hospital
1851 Paget resigns from post as Warden of the College and
      moves to Henrietta Street
1854 Paget appointed examiner to the East India Company
      John Snow completes his investigations during another
      epidemic of cholera
      Florence Nightingale becomes famous for her work in the
      Crimea
1857 Samuel Paget dies
1858 Paget moves to Harewood Place
1861 Paget appointed full surgeon to St Bartholomew's
      Hospital

1864 Pasteur proves that fermentation is caused by living
     organisms
1867 Lister publishes his historic paper on compound fractures
1871 Paget almost dies of infection acquired during the
     performance of a post-mortem examination
     Paget resigns from staff of St Bartholomew's Hospital
     Paget is made a baronet
1874 Paget publishes his paper on chronic ulceration of the
     nipple
1876 Paget publishes his first paper on osteitis deformans
     The Cruelty to Animals Act is passed
1877 Paget delivers the forty-ninth Hunterian Oration
1878 Paget gives up operating
1881 Paget presides over the Seventh International Congress
     of Medicine
1882 Robert Koch discovers the tubercle bacillus
1883 Koch discovers the bacterium responsible for cholera
1885 Pasteur succeeds in immunizing humans against rabies
1886 Paget appointed chairman of committee investigating
     control of rabies
1895 Death of Lydia Paget
1896 Paget completes work for the Royal Commission on
     Vaccination
1899 Death of James Paget

Preface

The second half of the nineteenth century was a period of rapid progress in British medicine, especially in the field of surgery. When seeking an explanation for this we tend to attribute it to a small number of key events, such as Simpson's introduction of surgical anaesthesia and Lister's control of wound infection. Further inquiry shows that these events provide only part of the explanation. Two additional elements contributed—firstly, the improvement in training of medical students, especially in physiology and pathology and, secondly, the emergence of the spirit of true professionalism among medical practitioners. It is with these two elements that the name of James Paget is linked.

Accurate diagnosis and effective treatment depend on an understanding of how the body functions in health and how it is altered by disease. John Hunter had given Britain the honour of leading the world in physiology and pathology, but after Hunter's death in 1793 this leadership passed to the Continent; French and German scientists made important discoveries, which for several decades went largely unheeded in Britain. Then in 1840 the young James Paget began to make a name for himself as a writer and teacher of physiology and pathology. His students caught his enthusiasm. A number of them became distinguished men of science; all were given an insight into the scientific basis of their vocation. No longer could they accept tradition and folk-lore as guides to diagnosis and treatment.

James Paget also influenced his students and colleagues in other ways. Both in his teaching and by his personal example he reminded them of their onerous responsibility to their patients. It was their duty to do their utmost, for as long as they remained in practice, to improve their knowledge and skill. Mistakes or failures could never be shrugged off as 'bad luck' or 'no worse than Dr X had done'; each must be carefully reviewed so that it could never happen again. He taught that there were to be no secrets kept from colleagues; medical knowledge should be shared, and acquired skills taught to others, so that all could benefit. Thus every practitioner should be both a teacher and a student for the whole of his career. He must also take great care that in his dealings with colleagues he was always honourable and courteous, since sharing of knowledge required mutual trust.

Thus he came to personify the new, thoroughly professional medical practitioner. Many a medical man faced with a problem asked himself, 'What would Sir James Paget do?' Many did, in fact seek his advice. Now it is nearly a century since his death. Medical science has made great strides, but human problems are much the same as they were during his lifetime. The principles that he established, both scientific and ethical, are as applicable to our times as they were to his.

In an account of the life of a medical man it is inevitable that a number of medical terms are used. Some of these require explanation. The word 'physic' was in common use until the mid-nineteenth century to denote that branch of medicine that deals with the treatment of disease of the internal organs by means of drugs and special diets. Its practitioners were known as 'physicians', a term that distinguished them from the surgeons and the apothecaries. In the twentieth century 'physic' has become 'internal medicine'. In Britain, and in some other English-speaking countries, specialists in this field are still known as 'physicians', but in the USA the term 'internist' is usually used. Confusion can also arise from the fact that 'physician' is sometimes applied to a practitioner of any branch of the profession; similarly, 'medicine' may mean 'internal medicine' or the whole range of practice. Fortunately, the meaning is usually clear from the context in which the terms occur.

'Clinical medicine' and 'clinical surgery' are terms used to denote those aspects of practice in which the physician or surgeon is dealing directly with individual patients. This form of practice is thus distinguished from laboratory investigational work and research.

'Physiology' is the study of the normal functioning of the organs and systems of the body. 'Pathology' is the study of disease processes and their effects on the structure and function of the body.

'Antiseptic' is an old term that was originally applied to a substance that prevented putrefaction. It came into common use after 1870, when it was applied to Lister's method of combating infection in surgical wounds. At first Lister aimed at killing bacteria that had already entered the wound. Later his technique was modified to prevent bacteria from gaining access. The process then became known as 'asepsis'.

Contents

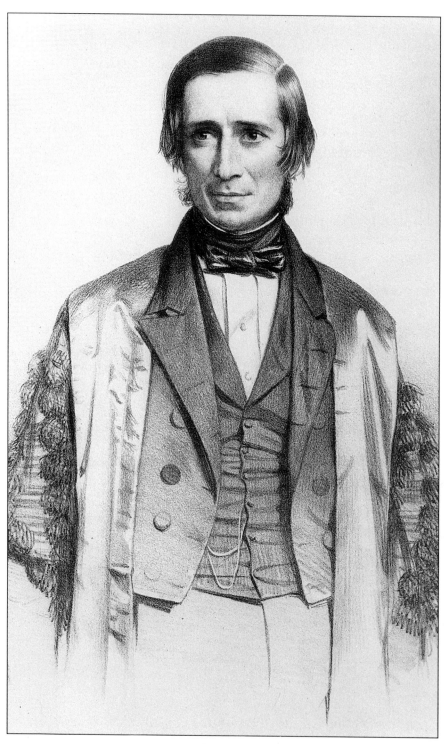

James Paget. Lithograph by TH Maguire, 1849. (Wellcome Institute).

Chapter 1

The House on the Quay

James Paget spent most of his life in London where, for forty years, he was a leader in the city's great medical and scientific institutions. But he was not a Londoner by birth. He was born in Great Yarmouth, Norfolk, on 11 January, 1814 and until he was twenty years old he had not travelled more than a few miles from his birthplace.

Great Yarmouth may have been provincial, but a growing lad would certainly not have found it dull. In the early years of the nineteenth century it was one of Britain's foremost commercial ports. Much of the nation's export trade in cotton goods and grain was channelled through Yarmouth, while ships from Scandinavia and Russia arrived there to discharge their cargoes of timber, iron, and pitch. A herring-fishing industry had flourished at Yarmouth since earliest times; each autumn, when the catch was at its peak, the local fishing boats were joined by hundreds more that came south from Scotland. The North Sea fleet of the Navy frequently used Yarmouth as its home port. It was to Yarmouth that Nelson returned in triumph after the Battle of the Nile, and to Yarmouth that the British wounded were brought after Waterloo. All these activities touched on the life of the Paget family and made lasting impressions on James and his brothers and sisters.

Alfred, the youngest of James's brothers, later recalled the Yarmouth of their childhood:

> The houses are well-built, not jerry-built. The old town, which merges into the new until even the new gains some mellowness, is full of unexpected charm; and the warm red roofs of the little cottages in the Rows catch at sunset an amazing wealth of colour. And Yarmouth has, what many seaside towns lack, a real work, a real profession, with the generous outgoings of the ships, and the labour on the Quays, and with the fishing vessels beating at evening into the Roads. Yarmouth lies north and south; along its eastern side is the sea, along its western the River Yare, broadening out towards the north into Breydon Water; over the river lie the South Town suburbs, and the two railway stations. To the south of the town the river joins the sea.
>
> Take your stand now on the old walls. Turn your back on the new town and the marine parade; you need not look on them to love Yarmouth. There below is the town. The spire of St Nicholas

stands up, and the tall masts of the ships in the river, and the smoking chimney of Lacon's brewery; but it is for the most part a low level of buildings. The last of those three or four streets, the one lying along the river, is the Quay, the straight line of merchants' houses, old and sweet smelling, some of them with oak ceilings and inner courts full of green leaves. And at your feet, cutting the streets right and left, even and crowded, are the Rows, paved alleys with the house doors of tiny houses on either side, most of them narrow, some only a few feet wide, some like Market Row wide enough to have good shops in them. They are neighbourly and they are old, and Yarmouth is seamed with them.

Yarmouth has never been unimportant; and it was always saved from mediocrity by its fishing. Now and then there were bad fishing years, 1817 was one and so was 1820; and the fishing was sometimes hindered by terrible storms which wrecked the sailing smacks. But as a rule the catches of mackerel and herring in the autumn were enormous, and made the town famous. From fishing the town won other renown for shipbuilding and for commerce: so that in 1830 it was the eighth port in England, and exceeding proud, with the only safe anchorage between the Thames and the Humber, trading in the Baltic and the Mediterranean, importing oak and pitch and tar, exporting corn and malt. If you were prosperous in Yarmouth, you became a shipowner.

Its communications in the early nineteenth century were as good as the times could make them. A mail coach travelled every day to and from the 'White Horse' in Fetter Lane via Ipswich, and a 'machine' went to Norwich twice a day in summer, once in winter. There was traffic by steambarges, wherries and carriers, and a coach three times a week to Gracechurch Street via Bury. The town was well-paved, well-lit, well-policed; the facts of poverty were kept decently in the background. It was hospitable to the last degree both to its neighbours and to its visitors; it was prosperous, self-satisfied, very kindly; it provided what the guidebooks of the time called 'a variety of elegant amusements'.

The jetty and the beach were the favourite promenades, and there was a racecourse on the South Denes. In 1788 a big public room was built at the north end of the Bath House, where tea and coffee were served morning and afternoon; London and local papers were to be seen, and Yarmouth met and gossiped with equal self-confidence over the latest bit of scandal or the possibility that the Corsican Wizard might foolishly make trouble in

Europe. Public breakfasts were held at the room, and occasional Balls and Parties: the subscription was only 10/- for a gentleman or 7/- for a lady.

In 1820 a Musical Festival was held at Yarmouth, and the account bears witness to the ambition of Yarmouth taste. A concerto for the flute and a Sonata for the harp were included in a ballad concert on the first day, and the local orchestra was helped by unprofessional musicians who were not allowed names on the programme. On the second day there was 'a Grand Selection of Sacred Music' at the Town Hall. On the third day the artists were still more grand, the composers still more miscellaneous. The programme promised 'The entire First Part of Haydn's celebrated Sacred Oratorio, The Creation; with two Grand Miscellaneous Acts selected from Mozart's Requiem. Beethoven's admired Sacred Oratorio called The Mount of Olives; Handel's Judas Maccabbeus and Israel in Egypt; with some highly esteemed compositions of Pergolese'. Among the stewards of this Festival was one Samuel Paget, a prosperous brewer of the town.[1]

Paget's father establishes the family business
Samuel Paget, the father of James and Alfred, had risen to his position of importance as the result of his own efforts. His ne'er-do-well father had given him only a meagre education and had taken no further interest in him. Fortunately, his mother was a woman of character who encouraged his ambitions. By reading, he educated himself to a standard that later enabled him to take his place with confidence among the leaders of the Yarmouth community. His first employment was as a clerk to a merchant who held a contract with the Admiralty for supplying provisions to Naval vessels. In 1791, when Samuel Paget was only seventeen, his employer died suddenly, leaving neither partner nor heir to carry on the business.

Samuel immediately travelled to London to present his credentials to the Admiralty. He had never visited the capital before. Its vastness and the crowds of people in the streets quite amazed him, but he quickly recovered his composure and at the Admiralty conducted himself with quiet confidence. He proved to the satisfaction of the officials that he had a sound knowledge of his late master's business. They agreed to transfer the contracts to him. Thus the young clerk became, at one stroke, the principal of his own firm.

With the support of his mother, who gave him her small savings, Samuel Paget was able to establish his business on a sound footing. In 1797 his association with a famous event in naval history enhanced his reputation. After the French invaded the Netherlands in 1795 they gave to a young Dutch officer, Jan de Winter, the task of rebuilding the Dutch navy. This de Winter did so well that two years later he was ready to attack the British North Sea fleet. The fleet was anchored in Yarmouth Roads when word was received that the Dutch had sailed. The British ships had to be made ready to put to sea at once. Samuel Paget supplied the necessary provisions and fresh water in record time. Under the command of Lord Duncan the North Sea fleet sailed into battle and won the notable victory of Camperdown. At the victory celebrations at Yarmouth Lord Duncan praised Paget and presented him with a gold medal.

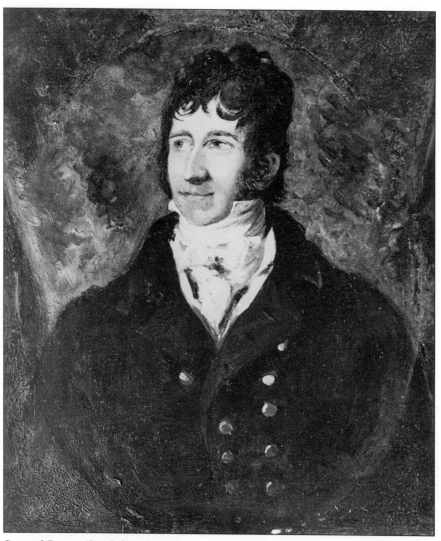

Samuel Paget. (Sir Julian Paget).

Samuel Paget marries Sarah 'Betsey' Tolver

In 1799, when he was twenty-five years old, Samuel Paget married. His bride was Sarah Elizabeth, the daughter of Mr Thomas Tolver of Chester. Tom Tolver was pleased to accept Samuel as a son-in-law, since it was apparent that young Paget was destined to succeed. Tolver had himself married a rich widow, by whom he had three daughters. Sarah, the eldest, was adopted by Tolver's sister,

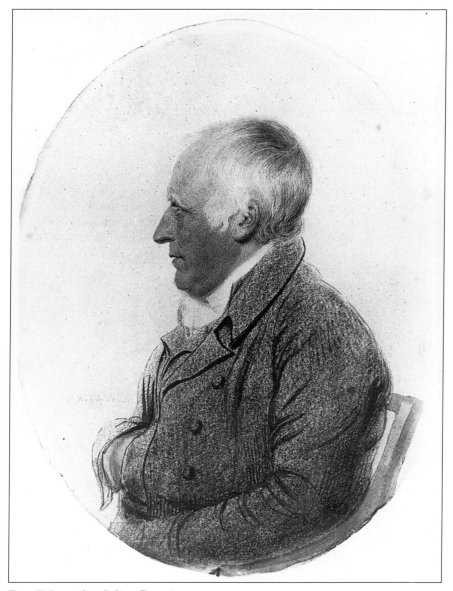

Tom Tolver. (Sir Julian Paget).

Mrs Godfrey. The Godfreys, who lived in Yarmouth, were childless but they proved to be excellent foster parents. They gave the little girl all the love and care she could need, and they also provided her with an education far superior to that usually thought suitable for females. Years later, Alfred, the youngest of Sarah Paget's sons, wrote:

> Martha Godfrey was handsome and rich, and she passed on to Sarah her fine discernment and her love of the arts. There is a little leather book of manuscript music in Sarah's writing, dated 1791 and traced with delicate care, where 'a lesson of Dr Handel' jostles with 'the Duke of York's Cotillion'. She passed on also an affection for independence and her own companionship.[2]

The Pagets were often amused by Tom Tolver. He saw himself as a sophisticated gentleman of fashion, whose duty it was to advise others on the finer points of etiquette. His wife's modest fortune enabled him to live comfortably without effort, so he had ample time to devote to these harmless pursuits. Tolver at first thought that one of his younger daughters would have made a better wife for Samuel Paget. In his view his eldest daughter's education had given her an unfortunate tendency to express opinions on serious matters and had made her altogether too domesticated for her future role as 'the leader and patroness among the ladies'. Despite Tom Tolver's misgivings, the marriage was a source of enduring happiness to both partners. James Paget had an explanation for his parents' devotion to each other:

> My mother was in some things very unlike him; and their marriage was a good example of that which seems a general rule—that the marriages are very happy in which those who are united are so far unlike that each may admire, in the other, qualities wanting in the self; and, with pride of ownership, may enjoy to see those qualities admired by others.[3]

In brief descriptions of his parents he hints at some of these differences:

> She was handsome, tall and graceful, somewhat hasty in temper, resolute, strong-willed and strong in speech . . .
> My father . . . was a rather small, active, handsome man; and I remember him in my boyhood as a good cricketer, a good speaker, gentle, calm, busy all day, and always seeming to love more than anything the quiet of his home.[4]

The young couple moved into a house on Yarmouth's South

Quay. On one side of this busy thoroughfare were the solidly-built houses of merchants and ship-owners. On the other side of the road, instead of houses, there was always a line of ships discharging or loading cargoes. The closeness of the houses on the Quay to the ships opposite was symbolic of the maritime interests of families like Samuel Paget's.

The business expands and diversifies

Paget worked diligently at expanding his business. Not content with provisioning vessels owned by others, he risked some of his hard-earned capital to buy ships of his own. Provided there were no disasters at sea, and the overseas markets had been correctly assessed, the venture could return handsome profits. But Samuel Paget was aware of the uncertainty of this type of enterprise and diversified his interests. In 1804, five years after his marriage, he became the senior partner in a brewery, which thereafter bore the name 'Paget and Company'. The brewery was to play an important role in the life of the family for more than forty years. It was one of Yarmouth's best known businesses and, among the breweries, it was second only to that owned by Sir Edmund Lacon.

The brewery flourished. In 1807 it was supplying no less than fifty-four public houses in Yarmouth and twenty-one in outlying areas. Profits rose from £1775 in 1805 to £3600 in 1810. The brewery became the mainstay of the family, but Samuel Paget retained his interest in shipping. As a loyal Yarmouth citizen, he was proud of the city's mercantile pre-eminence and eager to be associated with it. Furthermore, Englishmen were then living under the constant threat of invasion by the armies of Napoleon. They knew that their ships were the 'wooden walls' that kept the enemy at bay and maintained their trade links with the rest of the world. Patriotism, as well as personal inclination, led Samuel Paget to invest much of the profit from the brewery in merchant vessels.

Samuel and Betsey have a large family

Sarah Paget enthusiastically supported her husband in his business ventures, although domestic cares claimed much of her time and energy. Her first child, a daughter, was born in 1800. Within the family circle Sarah was always known as Betsey. The eldest daughter, christened Martha Maude, was given the pet-name of Patty. The Paget's first son was born a year later and was named Samuel. He died before he was two months old, his death being the first of many such sorrows to be experienced by the family. The second son, born in 1802, was also named Samuel, for it was not uncommon in those days to give the same name to a subsequent child when the first had died at an early age. This second son died when he was only four years old. In all, Betsey bore seventeen

children, of whom nine survived to adult life. This tragic record of
infant deaths was by no means unusual in nineteenth-century
families. Common childhood ailments, such as scarlet fever,
measles, and diphtheria were mainly to blame.

Between 1802 and 1811 four more children who were destined
to survive were added to the family—Frederick, born in 1805,
Arthur in 1808, George in 1809, and Charles in 1811. The original
home at 59, South Quay, was not large. Grandmother Paget lived

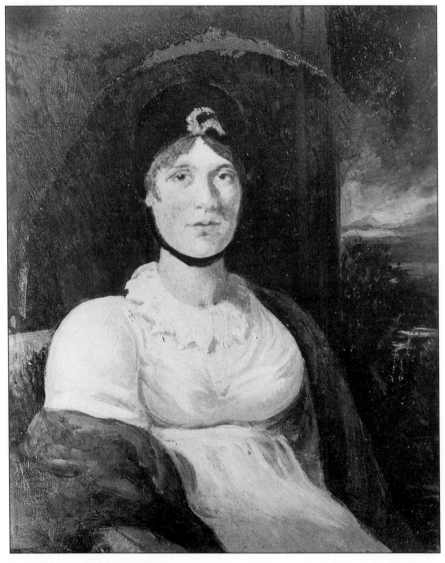

Betsey Paget. (Sir Julian Paget).

next door and a communicating passage was constructed between the two houses so that one of her rooms could be used as a nursery. But still more space was needed. In 1811 the family moved into temporary accommodation nearby, while the old home was demolished to make way for a new one.

A larger house is built

Although there were discomforts and inconvenience this was a happy time for Samuel Paget. He was prosperous and could take pleasure in providing for his family a new home that would be grander, as well as larger, than their previous one. A professional architect was engaged, but the eventual design owed as much to the family's friends and advisers as it did to him. Tom Tolver, with his eye for elegance, was responsible for the incorporation of a bow window in the dining room and for 'a large and handsome fanlight' in the passage. There were debates on such matters as the relative merits of stone and mahogany for the staircase. Samuel retained his composure and cheerfully despatched the cheques necessary to keep the builders at their work. He kept a record of the costs, totalling £7365-1-7, 'with the accuracy of the pence being equal to the importance of the pounds.'

The family moved into their new home at the end of 1813 and a month later James was born. Samuel Paget wrote in the family Bible 'James Paget, son of Samuel and Sarah Elizabeth Paget, Born

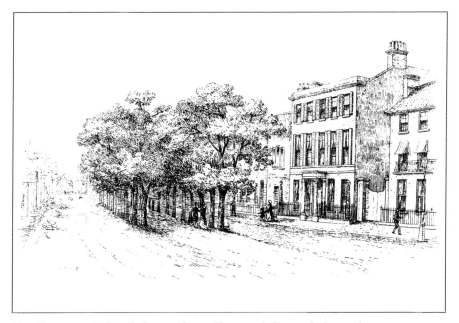

The House at 59, South Quay. (Great Yarmouth Borough Council.

11th January 1814, at 4 o'clock in the afternoon.' The father also wrote to his sister-in-law, Mrs Maria Moor, telling her of his wife's prolonged labour and expressing the hope that his family was now complete. However, five more children were born in the next eleven years. A boy and a girl died in infancy but three survived to adulthood—Francis, who was born in 1816, Alfred in 1818, and Katherine in 1825. Thus the eldest and the youngest of the children were the two girls, Patty and Kate, who were separated by an age difference of twenty-five years.

Civic duties and honours for Samuel Paget

The year 1814 was a successful one for Samuel Paget. He had been welcomed into the circle of Yarmouth's civic leaders and in October of that year he became an alderman. He was already an officer in the volunteer corps that had been formed to resist possible attacks by the French. He associated himself with several of the city's charitable organizations. In every way he was fulfilling Tom Tolver's expectation that he would succeed. Early in the year there were bright hopes of even better times ahead, since it seemed that the 'Corsican Wizard' had been driven from the stage of Europe forever. A great public celebration to mark 'the defeat of Napoleon and the Restoration of the Bourbons' was arranged for Tuesday, 9 April 1814. Samuel Paget was one of the principal organizers and Betsey his enthusiastic helper. Following a procession through the streets of the town there was a great outdoor banquet for rich and poor alike, at which roast beef and plum pudding were served, with beer to drink. Tables were set up end-to-end along the South Quay, the first table being outside the Pagets' home. The ladies of the neighbourhood were responsible for cooking and serving the food. Betsey had boiled in readiness thirty plum puddings of five pounds each. She later wrote to a relative, describing the events of the day:

> We roasted a rump of beef for the top and sent it in with a silk Union Jack. Every dish was covered, and though we furnished them with spoons, salt-spoon, etc., etc., nothing was lost nor was anything broken.[5]

The bands of the local militia paraded around the tables and provided music for the diners. Twenty toasts were drunk, including one to 'the speedy return of our townsmen imprisoned in France'. Betsey recalled:

> It is difficult to describe the emotion with which this toast was drunk: many hundreds of the Company had for years been mourning the captivity of husbands, fathers, sons, brothers and friends, whose return to their homes was, till this moment, more

hoped for than expected: suffice it to say that many, very many, drank it with tears of joy.[6]

At five o'clock the feast was terminated so that the revellers could enjoy donkey races on the Denes and the enormous bonfire that continued to blaze all night.

Never was such a day of harmony and unanimity witnessed; and it scarcely can be believed, but it is a positive fact, not one was seen in liquor.[7]

James was only three months old when this celebration was held. Nevertheless, as a child he heard his elder brothers describe it so often that he almost believed that he remembered the festivities himself. An occasion that he was just able to recall was that of 1817, when his father became Mayor of Yarmouth and a procession of aldermen in crimson robes marched to the house on the Quay to honour the new Mayor.

Samuel and Betsey guided their children by example

Samuel and Betsey were indulgent parents. They controlled the high spirits of their children without recourse to stern discipline. The example set by the parents themselves provided the children with a clear guide as to how they should order their lives. James wrote of his father:

I should give a very wrong impression of my father, if I were to speak of him only as a man of business. He was, in this, an admirable example; punctual, constant in work, perfectly fair, liberal and honest; even when he failed no one blamed him: but he was, besides, a thorough gentleman—cheerful, well-mannered, peace-loving, and hospitable; perfectly temperate, when frequent drunkeness was not deemed vile; refined in conversation even when cursing and nastiness were scarcely vulgar; and a lover of all that was simply beautiful in literature and art. Besides, he was a very active public-spirited man.[8]

Of his mother he wrote:

The qualities which one best remembers were her intense love of her children, her marvellous activity and industry, her admiration of all that was beautiful in art and nature, her skill in writing, needlework, and painting. She had seventeen children in twenty-six years: and nine of these, including the first born, grew up to full age. She took the close charge and guidance of them all: she managed all household affairs and, after the

manner of the time and place, did all the marketing and shop-
ping, directed the cookery, and made the choicest sweets. She
collected 'everything'—autographs, seals, and caricatures,
shells, corals and agates, old china and glass, and 'curiosities' of
all kinds—including all that she would induce the masters of my
father's ships to bring home from their long voyages; and all her
collections were orderly arranged and labelled in her own fair
hand . . .
In the midst of all this she was active in the society of the town:
hospitable, ready to do her share in all works of charity and
public amusements; and more than her share in politics, as a
thorough Tory with Mr Pitt for her hero. Besides, she took part,
even a leading and decisive part, in all grave business-questions;
and she was the most motherly of women. Of all her various
pursuits there was not one which she did not neglect or put aside
when one of her children was ill or unhappy, or on the point of
leaving home for any time or on his return from absence. Nor was
any of us ever absent but we had letters regularly with home
news and loving messages, and written in a handwriting so
beautiful as it is now very rare to find . . .
Such were my parents. I can boast of being, in the best sense,
well-born. The good qualities of the parents were transmitted
variously to the six brothers and two sisters among whom I grew
up. There was the same regard for home in all: especially among
those who remained there . . . One of the brothers was a thorough
entomologist: a sister more than maintained the autographs and
books of local history. Two were artists of rare skill; one of these,
an admirable writer; he left manuscript memoirs of three of his
brothers, written as commentaries on collections of their letters.
They might have been published as romances of real life. And in
all the family there was not one who did not show power and
strong will for work; not one who was ever unfair, stupid, or
dishonest.[9]

The boys all attended a little local school, which James describes
in his memoirs:

It was kept by Mr Bowles, a careful, well-mannered, and generally well-informed man, who had been an actor and now was
minister of the Unitarian Chapel. I have an impression that the
greater part of the private schools in small towns at that time
were kept by persons who had failed in other callings in life, and
who were generally deemed unfit for the public service or any
more active business. Religious teaching was not commonly
much thought of; if it was wished for, parents at home gave it: at
least, they did who were as simply pious as mine were, though

the teaching seldom went beyond the Church Catechism and the influence of good example. The education at Mr Bowles's was not of a very high order; neither was it accurate or profound or of a kind likely to encourage deeper study. In the highest class it went as far as quadratic equations, the first six books of Euclid, and to undefined distances in Horace and Virgil, after Caesar and Sallust; and in Homer, after Xenophon and a Greek Delectus. In all these there was little more to be done than oral translation and parsing in classes; there was but little attempt at composition or verse-writing, and very little of history, geography, or the use of the globes. Still, it seems to have been a very fair education for what it cost—eight guineas a year; and it was given punctually and carefully and with sufficient penalties for negligence.[10]

Less is known about the education of the two girls, Patty and Kate. Lessons given by their mother were probably supplemented with tuition in drawing and music by visiting teachers, such as John Crome, the famous landscape painter. The mother was the most talented artist in the family and it was from her that the boys inherited their 'rare skill'. A pencil sketch 'Woolsey's Mill, Near Yarmouth' made by James when he was a young man bears witness to his ability. James also played the flute and sang, although he did not take his musical activities very seriously. The varied talents and the energy of the Paget children ensured that their home life

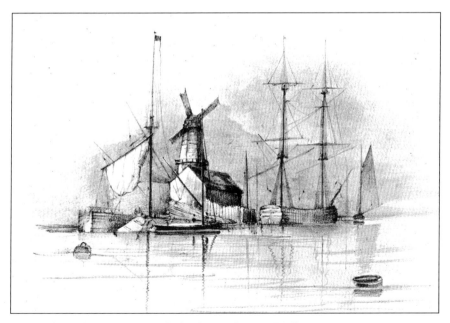

Woolsey's Mill Near Yarmouth, by James Paget. (Wellcome Institute).

was never dull. They encouraged and stimulated each other. Their wholehearted sharing of success and failures forged bonds of loyalty that lasted all their lives.

The children were fond of staging their own theatrical performances to celebrate special occasions, such as 11 January, which was

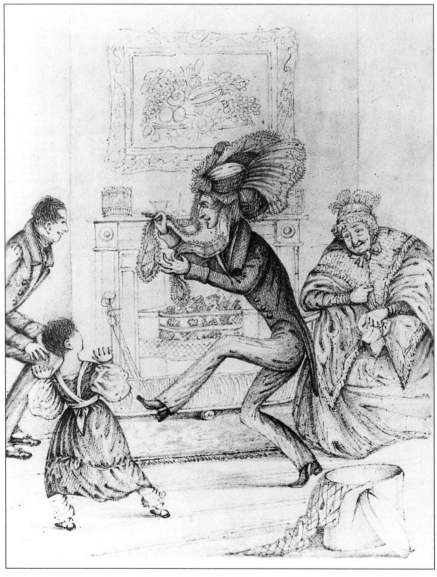

Miss Carrington's Cap. A drawing by Charles Paget; it shows George imitating a lady of their acquaintance for the amusement of James, Kate and Grandmamma Paget. (Sir Julian Paget).

the birthday of both James and Alfred. In 1830, when James turned sixteen and Alfred twelve, they started rehearsals several days before the event. They improvised a stage with curtains and concocted costumes for the boys by dividing between them the components of Samuel Paget's carefully preserved military uniform. All went well until the finale, when actors and audience were all overcome with laughter. Alfred later recalled the happy mood of that evening:

> Verily, good cheer seemed imperishable; and to me or James, whose birthdays came on the same day, it seemed as if a double portion remained to the youngest. Charles and George will never go to bed while there is a good story still to tell, after James has sung his song of The Legacy, or Tom Bowling, till we cry again. It was not the words, I say in excuse, 'twas the voice: 'twas a note or two of his that even now have a moving power in one of his speeches upon a family occasion. George and Charles and Arthur and James—long after I am or ought to be asleep there they are still on the landing, laughing and joking and answering again, till my sister has her opinion of the waste of candles, and the house seems as if it would never break up or go to bed.[11]

Such family occasions were frequently attended by Grandmother Paget, who would sit in her comfortable armchair, smiling quietly at the frolics of the children. Charles has drawn her in just this attitude as she watches George cavorting about in disrespectful imitation of a grand lady who was well known to them all. Sometimes the Pagets were joined by Tom Tolver, or by Betsey's sisters, Aunts Moor and Bagnall. Samuel Paget had many friends and business associates to whom he often extended hospitality, but the family was largely self-sufficient. When there was a family occasion to be celebrated outsiders were not needed.

The children were not sheltered from knowledge of the serious matters that occupied their parents' attention. From the windows of their home they could observe the arrivals and departures of ships owned by their father. Pleasure at a safe homecoming could be quickly destroyed by the news of another ship being lost at sea, sometimes with the deaths of local men who had been good friends for many years. For the children the fact that many of the ships bore names of members of the family heightened the poignancy. But even more than the ships, the brewery entered into the daily life of the family.

The brewery was at the North End. Between it and the house was the whole length of the Quay, with the pleasant respectable houses of the Yarmouth gentry. Each stone was familiar, with a pretty bit of scandal or a little bitterness of rivalry or a sudden glowing of friendship. Day by day, year by year, the life of the Pagets flowed and ebbed between the Brewery and Home. There were few distractions from the direct way of the Quay—here was enough for adventure and education. You will never be intimate with the Pagets if you belittle the Brewery or think of it only as a useful trade or as a source of income. Think of it rather as something wonderfully loved, as a vocation demanding sacrifice, as the very proof of hard work and honesty, as that which must at all cost be saved for the children. The children grew to reverence it and spelled its name always with a capital 'B'.[12]

The Paget boys' education

Each of the three eldest boys, on reaching the age of thirteen, was taken from Mr Bowles's establishment and sent to the famous Charterhouse School in London. Samuel Paget had given the matter careful thought. His opinions on the subject of education for boys were expressed in a letter he wrote to a widowed relative who had sought his advice with regard to her own son.

I am not one of those who feel disposed to let them follow what profession or trade they *think* they like, unless I consider it myself eligible. But at the same time, as it not infrequently happens, that when the mind of a boy shows a *bias,* it at one and

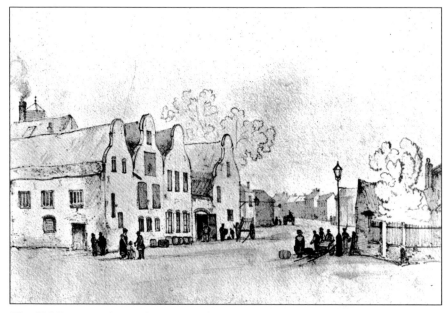

The Old Brewery. A pencil sketch by Charles Paget. (Sir Julian Paget)

the same instant shows also a sort of talent or aptitude to attain one particular trade or profession more than another, I should under circumstances like these be disposed to avail myself of such favourable impression by letting that be a boy's pursuit.[13]

He went on to say that 'a couple of years in a good school gives . . . an uncommon advantage to a young man as he advances in life . . .' Accordingly, Frederick, Arthur, and George all became pupils at Charterhouse. Frederick seems to have profited less from his schooling than his father had hoped. The other two boys were more successful. Arthur's teachers thought him an excellent scholar; George was unusual in having an aptitude for mathematics in an age when most boys studied only the classics. Consequently, George won prizes in mathematics, while being considered sound but not brilliant in his other subjects.

The success of these two boys at Charterhouse prompted their father to extend himself still further on their behalf. Both went on to Cambridge, Arthur to prepare himself for a career in law, George still undecided as to his ultimate vocation.

The next son, Charles, did not follow in the footsteps of his elder brothers. His health was so poor that he could not go away to school. He was educated at home and was to join his father in the family business.

Financial restraints prevent James entering Charterhouse
By the time a decision had to be made about the education of James, Samuel Paget was faced with problems of a different kind. The years of prosperity that had followed the peace of 1815 were over. Yarmouth was losing its pre-eminence as a commercial port. The Navy was reduced to peacetime strength, so contracts for the provisioning of the North Sea fleet came to an end. But the most important factor was the change in Samuel Paget himself. The youth who had shown such initiative had grown into a cautious, less imaginative middle-aged man. He had allied himself with business partners who only added to his anxieties and contributed nothing to the profitability of the joint enterprise. A number of his investments in ships had proved disastrous, so he sold the rest of them. Increasingly grave financial problems were to be a dominant factor in the life of the family for decades to come. One of the early consequences was that the father who had so delighted in providing well for his family had to deny the younger sons the benefits of public school education. James continued at Mr Bowles's school until he was sixteen. In later life he commented:

I have no doubt that I thus suffered heavy loss. I learned as much as I could, and for the last year or more was the head boy in the school; and I did my best in after years to increase my 'school-learning' ; but I never could acquire anything fairly to be called classical knowledge: I could translate enough for the commonplace understanding of a Latin or Greek book, but never could acquire any classic taste or enjoy the influence of any ancient writer, or take part in any of the learned table-talk to which in later years I was admitted—unless it were that most popular of parts, the part of a listener who appeared intelligent. Equal, or perhaps greater, was the loss in the fitness or the facility for social life; but how great this was I cannot judge, or how far I showed the defects which I have so often heard attributed to those who have not enjoyed the advantages of public schools and universities.[14]

James's career is chosen

Towards the end of his schooldays James thought he would like to go into the Navy. There was much to commend this choice to his father: '. . . the Navy was at least a profession for a gentleman; the education for it was very cheap and my father had friends in it.' So during his last year of schooling James studied navigation and had extra lessons in mathematics. Just before he turned sixteen his father wrote a letter to an old friend, Captain Sir Eaton Travers, requesting that he arrange for James's entry into the Navy. The request would most probably have been granted. Samuel Paget set out to deliver the letter personally, but had last-minute misgivings. He reached Sir Eaton's doorstep but then turned back; next day he burned the letter. James was at first disappointed, but soon came to realise that his father had acted wisely. The prospect of adventure and the glamour of a smart uniform had for a time blinded the boy to the fact that he was not temperamentally suited to the life of a naval officer.

James does not record how he and his parents made their final decision as to his vocation. By whatever means the decision was made, it was acted upon on 9 March, 1830. On that date documents were signed, binding James Paget to spend five years as an apprentice to learn 'the art and mystery of a Surgeon and Apothecary.'

Chapter 2

The Apprentice Surgeon-Apothecary

In 1830 there were several routes by which a young man could enter the medical profession; he chose the one that best matched his ambition and his father's pocket. If he aimed to be a physician he would first need to complete his education at a university, since the Royal College of Physicians of London required this proof that he was well versed in the classics and possessed 'perfect Latinity'. An Oxford or Cambridge degree would qualify him for the College's Fellowship. If, on the other hand, he had attended a Scottish or Irish university, he would have to be content with the more lowly Licence of the College. Licentiates greatly outnumbered Fellows, but only Fellows were eligible for election to the Council, the governing body of the College. Having completed his university studies the student spent a year at a hospital, attending lectures and accompanying senior physicians on their visits to the wards. He then took examinations in physic (internal medicine); the examinations were usually conducted in Latin.

Physicians advised and treated patients suffering from internal disorders. Medical knowledge had not advanced to a stage where diagnosis was often possible, even for the wisest practitioners, so they took detailed histories and prescribed medicines for the relief of symptoms. The physicians' prescriptions were dispensed by apothecaries, who were much lower in the medical social scale, but greatly outnumbered their more learned colleagues.

An apothecary acquired his skill by a five-year apprenticeship in an apothecary's shop. Here he became familiar with the drugs in common use, and learned how to dispense the complicated medicines that were then in vogue. His training also included lectures in physic. Hence apothecaries believed that they were capable of prescribing, as well as dispensing, but so that they would not encroach on the territory of physicians, they were not permitted to charge for both services; if they were paid for their advice they could not also ask payment for the medicine they supplied. Their training and certification were controlled by the Society of Apothecaries, which issued its Licence to candidates who met its requirements.

Surgeons also received their vocational training as apprentices. Their choice of a master very largely determined the pattern of their subsequent careers. An able young man apprenticed to an eminent London surgeon could look forward to entering consulting practice, once he had completed his apprenticeship and passed the examination for the Membership of the Royal College of Surgeons of London. His private patients would be rich and generous, but he would also hold an appointment at a large hospital where he would treat the poor for the rewards of personal satisfaction and enhanced professional reputation. Good apprenticeships were expensive, the usual fee being five hundred pounds, although some apprentices were accepted on more favourable terms if there were family ties or friendships to recommend them.

James becomes an apprentice general practitioner

Young men who could not afford a London apprenticeship could obtain their training with a surgeon in a provincial town or country district for a much smaller fee. If they were able to live at home while studying the cost was reduced still further. At the completion of their apprenticeship they took the examination for the Membership of the Royal College of Surgeons, but few of them would become consulting surgeons. Apprentices of provincial surgeons usually became general practitioners like their masters. For this type of practice a dual qualification, combining the Membership of the Royal College of Surgeons with the Licence of the Society of Apothecaries, was considered appropriate. Indeed, the old title of 'surgeon-apothecary' was just being replaced by that of 'general practitioner' when James Paget became an apprentice. An able and hard-working general practitioner would be a respected member of his community and, in time, would earn a reasonable income, but it was unlikely that he would ever achieve professional distinction. (A notable exception was Edward Jenner. Jenner had been apprenticed to a surgeon at Sodbury in Gloucester and was a general practitioner at Berkeley when he became famous for his work on vaccination against smallpox. However, as a young man he had worked as an assistant to John Hunter for two years; a friendship between the two was maintained by correspondence until Hunter's death twenty years later. Jenner was thus not working in isolation in his country village, but was stimulated by his association with one of the greatest scientists of the age.)

Paget's apprenticeship would prepare him for general practice. His surgical qualification would vouch for his competence to perform amputations, set broken bones, and to carry out the small range of operations that constituted the repertoire of the country or provincial surgeon. It also permitted him to bleed patients, to treat skin ailments, and to give treatment for any other abnormal conditions that appeared on the surface of the body. As an apothecary he would be able to prescribe and dispense medicines for the relief of symptoms of internal disease. This part of his training would also make him neat and accurate in his handling of drugs, and business-like in the keeping of accounts, for the apothecary was still a shop-keeper, although a rising generation of general practitioners was seeking improved professional status.

The usual period of apprenticeship was five years but, in James's case, it was to be reduced to four and a half years, the last part of his training being obtained at one of the large London hospitals. Perhaps his father thought that this would be a small compensation for his missing the experience of attending a university.

James began his apprenticeship with joyous enthusiasm. He was just sixteen years old, but he seems to have sensed almost at once that henceforth medicine would dominate his life. The realisation was accompanied by a change in his personality. His memoirs and the family chronicles suggest that, as a child, he was somewhat overshadowed by his more exuberant brothers. Arthur, we are told, was handsome, clever, and endowed with great personal charm. George we glimpse as a sound student and an entertaining companion. The younger brothers' artistic ability won them praise. James seems to have stayed quietly in the background, playing a supporting role. But when he began his apprenticeship he discovered that he, too, had special talents. His diffidence was replaced by the confidence of one who senses that he is at the beginning of a notable career.

James's master was a general practitioner-surgeon of Great Yarmouth, Mr Charles Costerton. Costerton's practice was not the largest in the town but he was held in high regard. He had been Mayor of Yarmouth in 1825. He knew the Paget family well, having treated Charles Paget on a number of occasions. He usually had several apprentices, the most senior of whom would normally have given James his first instruction. However, in 1830 James was Costerton's only apprentice, so he had the good fortune to be taught personally by the master, whom he liked and respected. James later recalled:

> The necessary daily work was dull, and at times tedious and apparently useless. One had to be in the surgery from about 9 to 1, and again (I think) from 2 or 3 to 5 or 6, every day; and there one's time was chiefly occupied in dispensing, seeing a few outpatients, as they might be called, of the poorer classes, in receiving messages, making appointments, keeping accounts, and at Christmas-time making-out bills, and, for some, receiving payments. When the master came in from his rounds of visits, one had to write, at his dictation, for each day—*Die Lunae, Die Martis, Die Jovis,* or whatever god it might be—the name of each patient he had seen, the fact of the *Visitatio,* and the prescription of the medicines required. Then these were to be made-up and sent; the bottles to be neatly corked and covered; the pills to be duly rolled and smoothly rounded (no silvering then), the leeches

to be put in their boxes with scarcely struggling-room; and all to look as neat as from any druggist's shop. And from this book were duly entered in another the supplies of time and physic, and the cost of each for each patient. I was taught and soon learned to do all this by Mr Costerton himself.[1]

The opportunities for learning extended beyond these 'broom and apron' aspects of apprenticeship. The patients who consulted Mr Costerton provided a good introduction to general practice. Not all of them were seriously ill:

Among the outpatients (as I called them) were ulcerated legs, useful for bandaging, and coughs and colds, and occasional slight injuries; and not a few, especially women, who came to be bled. For at that time there were not a few, especially among the country working-people, who deemed bleeding once or twice a year a great safeguard, or a help to health. They came frequently on market-days at the time of spring and fall, and generally did their day's work in the market and then walked to the surgery. There they were at once bled, and usually were bled till they fainted, or felt very faint and became pale; then a pad was put over the wounded vein, and a bandage round the elbow; and they went home, often driving three or four miles into the country. I have no recollection of any evidence that either good or harm was ever done by this practice.[2]

In the notes he made of his first major case James records the horrors of surgery before the advent of anaesthesia.

A young boatman was pushing off his boat, over the bow of which was one of the big swivel-guns then in common use for shooting wild-fowl as they flew in flocks low over the snow or ice. An accidental pull at the trigger fired the gun, and the great charge of big shot went through the inner half of the poor fellow's left knee- and elbow-joints. Both limbs were amputated. He bore the operations very bravely (there was no use of ether or chloroform then), and I bore the sight of the amputation of the thigh; but, when the first intense occupation of the mind in curiosity was over, there seemed more opportunity for sympathy, and at the amputation of the arm I was very faint, and had to stand aside, useless.[3]

James recognises the ineptness of many practising surgeons

As he became more experienced James was able to assist his master in a number of surgical operations. He was also invited to watch the work of other surgeons in the town. He soon perceived that there was a wide variation in the technical skills of these different operators. He had a high regard for his master's ability, but there were others from whom he learned by witnessing their demonstrations of ineptness.

Costerton taught him the anatomy of the skeleton and supervised his dissecting of the internal organs of cadavers. From time to time additional tuition was available:

> ... In my second year I was able to attend a course of lectures on the bones, given by Mr Randall, a young surgeon who had then just settled for practice at the village of Acle, about ten miles from Yarmouth. They were given in a room at the Angel Inn in the market-place, the class consisting of some six or eight pupils of surgeons in the town. I have full notes of them, and as I read them now they seem at least as good as could have been derived from any demonstrations or lectures on anatomy in a first-year's study in a London school at that time.[4]

These 'full notes' are at present in the library of the Royal College of Surgeons, London. They consist of scores of pages of fine, neat handwriting, with scarcely an alteration; they were probably written from notes taken during the lectures.

James's reading extended to a range of standard works on internal medicine, as well as the works of the leading writers on surgery.

> I read, I believe, the whole of Mason Good's 'Study of Medicine', and all Cullen's 'Practice of Physic', and much of his 'Materia Medica'. I read, also, the courses of lectures by Abernethy, Astley Cooper, and Lawrence, published in the 'Lancet', and Thompson's 'Lectures on Inflammation'; all the papers in the 'Cyclopaedia of Medicine', then in course of publication, all the current numbers of the 'Lancet', and many more books, from which, probably, I learned little more than the art of reading quickly.[5]

A little further on he comments unfavourably on some of the forms of treatment he saw being used:

> It is hard to remember anything of the methods of practice then generally used, which is still instructive; for observations on the effects of treatment were vaguely made, not exactly recorded, not tabulated; and the principles were deemed sure, whatever consequences might ensue from observance of them. Yet, from some parts of the practice, one may still derive instruction.[6]

It is not clear whether these are the judgements of the mature writer of the memoirs or of the young apprentice. Probably the doubts he had in his youth were clarified in retrospect by the great scientific advances of the second half of the century.

Britain's first cholera epidemic

One of the events of medical history he witnessed during his apprenticeship was Britain's first cholera epidemic. The outbreak began in 1826, in India, from where it spread westwards into Europe, reaching Russia in 1830 and Germany two years later. The disease is thought to have been brought to the eastern ports of Britain by German sailors. The cause of cholera was still unknown; the medical profession distinguished it from other diseases associated with diarrhoea simply on the basis of its greater severity and high mortality. Before the nineteenth century ended, three different branches of science contributed to the understanding and control of cholera. Engineers prevented epidemics by providing safe water supplies and efficient sewerage systems; microbiologists identified the cholera bacterium, thus providing a basis for accurate diagnosis; and physicians recognised that dehydration, which could often be corrected, was the commonest cause of death in cholera victims.

This last feature of the disease was beginning to attract interest in 1832, as Paget indicates:

I saw many cases of it, and saw them vainly treated—some with bleeding, some with calomel and opium, some with saline injections into the veins—all uselessly, though I can still remember the surprising and misleading revival of a woman who, while the saline injection was going-on, was roused from an apparently impending death in the cold blue collapse, and sat up and talked, and for an hour or two seemed quite revived.[7]

The patient's failure to survive suggests that the volume of fluid used was insufficient.

Frederick leaves home

Meanwhile, the pattern of family life in the house on the Quay was changing. In 1831 Frederick decided to marry. Since leaving school he had worked in the family business and had been made a partner. Now that he needed capital to set up a home, it was necessary for him to relinquish his partnership and take cash in lieu; this added to his father's financial problems. The young couple made their home in Yarmouth, where Frederick had obtained employment in a bank, but the wife died less than three years after the marriage. Frederick left Yarmouth, hoping to improve his prospects, and for

some years he lived in Europe. He remarried and had a family, but
was always short of money. His father helped him whenever he
could. Of all Samuel Paget's children, this eldest son was the one
least conscious of the bonds of family affection.

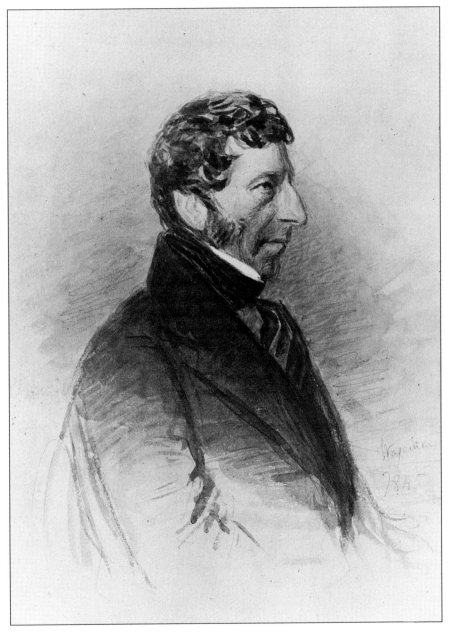

Frederick Paget. (Sir Julian Paget).

George excels at Cambridge

Although times were bad, there were still occasions for celebration in the house on the Quay. George was studying for his degree at Caius College, Cambridge. The family had always considered him to be competent and industrious, but not brilliant. Thus they were

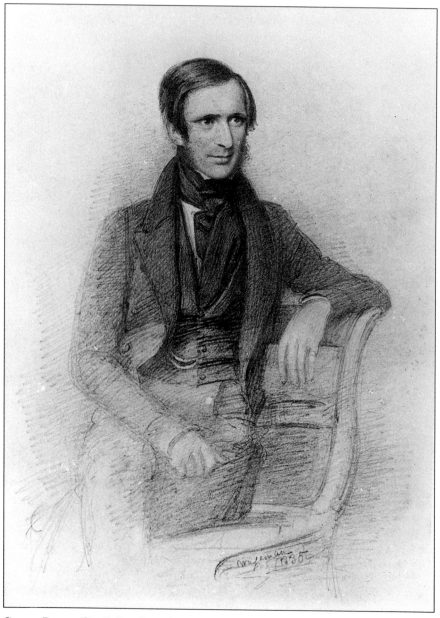

George Paget. (Sir Julian Paget).

surprised and delighted to learn that George Paget was highly placed in the mathematics Honour List for 1831; he was grouped with some distinguished scholars. Samuel Paget wrote to George:

> I will not attempt to describe the pleasure, the unspeakable pleasure, your letter has given me and your dear mother, whose heart has been, all the week, so full of the deepest anxiety ... your letter was given me in bed this morning, the parcels of the Bury coach not being delivered till the morning. In ten minutes the whole house was uproarious, and you may easily conceive the delight of all. Charles and James said it was worth reading a whole life, to have such an hour of rejoicing.[8]

A year later there was even better news from Cambridge. George was elected to a Fellowship. The terms of the Fellowship required the holder to be a Norfolk man and studying for the medical profession. So George's vocation was decided. He would begin the study of physic, anatomy, and chemistry under the guidance of Cambridge lecturers, Drs Haviland, Clark, and Cumming. Samuel Paget now had two sons preparing to be doctors, but the prospects of the two young men were very different. George's Cambridge degree would be followed by a Fellowship of the Royal College of Physicians, while James's course of study would lead to a provincial general practice. James's professional and social status would be much lower than his brother's.

Of greater practical importance to the parents was the fact that George's Fellowship was well endowed. Not only would he be self-supporting, but he would also be able to help with the educational expenses of his younger brother. It was with thankfulness, as well as pride, that Betsey wrote her congratulations to George:

> How am I to express myself for what I am to say? Good God, never can I express our delight and astonishment, when we (that is your dear father, Charles and myself with Kate) opened your letter in the Post Office Row. May we ever with humble thankfulness praise Him who has showered such blessings upon us. We instantly ran to Frederick's whose joy was equal to our own. A bottle of best sherry was broached and your health and continued success drank in a bumper. Then we came home to communicate the extraordinary intelligence to Patty, etc., and we certainly obeyed your orders in ringing as loud as the day would allow us, (you know it was Sunday).[9]

Arthur's career falters and his health declines

While George had exceeded his family's expectations, Arthur's scholastic career had been disappointing. A popular young man, he had been too easily drawn into the social life of the university and had neglected his studies. Arthur left Cambridge without any academic distinction to promote his entry into the legal profession. The healthy self-esteem, which had led him as a schoolboy to refer to himself as 'the future Lord Chancellor', was waning. While living in shabby rooms in London he began, at the age of twenty-three, to experience bouts of depression and loneliness. His unhappiness was intensified when he fell deeply in love, but the lady spurned his proposal of marriage.

In the same year, 1831, he went into Chambers at the Temple. His work as a barrister now required him to go on Circuit. When he was in Yarmouth the family noticed that he was irritable and seemed unwell. They ascribed this to the stress of work, combined with anxiety over money. But in November, 1833, his condition was diagnosed as consumption. His physician advised him to move to the south coast where, he hoped, rest and the warmer climate would prove beneficial. But Arthur's health was deteriorating rapidly. He was too sick to undertake the journey and had to appeal to his parents for help. Samuel Paget came to London at once and was greatly alarmed at the condition of his son. With his father's help the invalid managed to make the journey home by stage coach.

Once at home he was lovingly cared for, but his sickness made him impatient and moody. The only attendant he could tolerate was his brother James. Patty wrote in her journal:

> From James he would bear almost anything and appeared to lean completely on him. Was it not singular, wonderfully singular, that he should, poor fellow, persevere in coming downstairs on the Christmas day? He walked downstairs by 10 in the morning . . . He would have James place the easy chair in the dining room and soon to dinner did we sit down. He ate a nice dinner, some turkey and a small piece of mutton and took a glass of wine. He remained with us till seven, when he said he was rather tired, and then walked upstairs and went to bed. Thus remained faithful the son to whom above all others, home was home and the family traditions, the Christmas cheer, the toasts in Malmsey were rites to be observed at all cost.[10]

Early the next morning Arthur died. His death was a crushing blow to a family already struggling against adversity.

James becomes a self-taught botanist

James was fortunate that he did not contract his brother's disease. He returned to his medical studies and became engrossed in a new project—a study of the plant life of the region. In his memoirs he describes how his career as a botanist began:

My mother's love of collecting had influenced in various degrees all her children; chiefly, in relation to natural history, my next elder brother Charles and myself. He gave himself chiefly to entomology; I to botany, being guided to it by Mr Palgrave, a nephew of Mr Dawson Turner, who represented in Yarmouth what might justly be called the Norfolk School of Botanists. Its leader had been Sir James Smith, the purchaser of the Linnaean collections and chief founder of the Linnaean Society; and now its chief members were Mr Turner and his son-in-law Sir William Hooker.

I cannot remember all the times at which I used to collect. I think they were chiefly on Saturday afternoons, and on casually unoccupied bits of days, and often before breakfast, when I would gather algae on the beach, and the plants which were abundant on the Denes and sand-cliffs and salt-marshes near the town, and were valuable for exchange with inland collectors. They were enough to enable me to make a nearly complete collection of the Flora of the district, with specimens for exchange with other botanists, especially with the Hookers and some of their pupils, and with Coterell Watson.... I studied the botany of the district sufficiently to take part with my brother Charles in publishing the *Natural History of Great Yarmouth;* a thin 8vo in which I first appeared in print. He supplied the entomological part of it, I the rest, using not merely my own collections but those of all the local naturalists who had recorded anything within my reach of their observations. The enumeration of species was, I think, nearly complete for that time. It would be more than complete for the present time; for drainage and various cultivations, including even that of Natural History itself, have sadly exterminated many of the species we used to be proud of.[11]

There was a practical objective, as well as a love of science, prompting the two brothers to produce their book—they hoped it would earn some money. Its full title was *A Sketch of the Natural History of Yarmouth and its Neighbourhood, containing Catalogues of the Species of Animals, Birds, Reptiles, Fish, Insects and Plants, at present known. By CJ and James Paget, Yarmouth. F Skill, 1834.* It sold for half-a-crown. The 32-page introduction written by James, was followed by 88 pages of catalogue, in which were described 766 insects and 1185 plants. The Natural History was published shortly after James finished his apprenticeship with Charles Costerton. It sold well and, despite its modest price, returned a useful profit to its authors.

James the earnest apprentice may have had some doubts as to the wisdom of devoting so much time to his botanical interests. (An old lady had said that the young man could hardly be a serious student of medicine since he was constantly to be seen walking about Yarmouth!) But in later life, when he reflected on this period, he was certain it had not been a mistake:

> I think it impossible to estimate too highly the influence of the study of botany on the course of my life. It introduced me into the society of studious and observant men; it gave me an ambition for success, or at the worst some opportunities for display in subjects that were socially harmless; it encouraged the habit of observing, of really looking at things and learning the value of exact descriptions; it educated me in habits of orderly arrangement. I can think of none among the reasons of my success—so far as I can judge of them—which may not be thought-of as due in some degree to this part of my apprentice-life. My early associations with scientific men; my readiness to work patiently in museums, and arrange them, and make catalogues; the unfelt power of observing and of recording facts; these and many more helps towards happiness and success may justly be ascribed to the pursuit of botany.

> And, as I look back, I am amused in thinking that of the mere knowledge gained in the study—the knowledge of the appearences and names and botanical arrangement of plants—none had in my after-life any measure of what is called practical utility. The knowledge was useless: the discipline of acquiring it was beyond all price.[12]

Paget's other interests

Botany was not the only non-medical subject he found time to study. He improved his knowledge of Latin and Greek and also taught himself to read French well enough to be able to translate scientific texts. Thus he prepared his own translations of Bichat's *Anatomie Generale* and *Sur la Vie et la Mort*. He translated Cuvier's classification of the animal kingdom and fixed it to the wall of his bedroom so that he could memorize it while dressing. He repeated some of the famous basic experiments of chemistry and for a time considered extending his studies in science. His interests also ranged beyond the purely scientific; he decided to join his brothers Charles and Alfred in their drawing lessons:

> 'Young Crome' succeeded 'Old Crome' in his weekly visits at the house, and nearly all of us had lessons from him. Two of my brothers, Charles and Alfred, might have lived as artists, such skill had they; I had very little; yet it was enough to enable me to learn to make sketches of scenery and of some of the simpler

objects of natural history, and even of pathological specimens.
Some of these are in the Hospital collection; a fungus haema-
todes, and an ulcerated caecum—with which I remember that
the widow of the patient was so charmed that she begged for a
copy of it. I wonder whether this is now in the possession of her
distinguished grandson.

I may repeat concerning this meagre education of a little artistic
skill and taste nearly what I have said of botany. Its immediate
utility was too little, its indirect utility too great, to be told. It
helped to enable me to look and see more in things than some
could see; it strengthened the power of remembering things seen;
it made it easy to illustrate my lectures with sketches which I
could describe while making them; and it helped to give me such
a love of scenery and of pictures that I have never once regretted
my having been unable to learn any one of the sports or active
games which to some seem essential to the happiness of a
holiday.[13]

The remaining family at Yarmouth

Despite his numerous personal interests James was conscious of
the family's shared anxieties. With Frederick's marriage, Arthur's
death, and George's absence at Cambridge, those who remained in
the house on the Quay were becoming even more closely dependent
on each other. Charles and Frank, the brothers closest in age to
James, had joined the family firm, from necessity as much as choice.
Their father could not have continued to conduct the brewery
without their help. Charles was the firm's accountant, Frank
supervised the workmen.

These two brothers were very different personalities. The elder,
Charles, was thoughtful and serious. He brooded over their business problems and could escape from his worries only when he was
able to turn his attention to his hobby, entomology; as he bent over
his collection of butterflies his frown would be replaced by a smile.
Frank was energetic and cheerful. He set about each day's work at
the brewery with eagerness; once finished, he would enjoy an
evening stroll along the Quay, his mind at ease. Neither Charles
nor Frank enjoyed good health. Charles suffered from chronic
infection (osteomyelitis) of a thigh bone. He was never entirely free
from pain and from time to time the condition flared up, necessitat-
ing agonising operations to drain the infected bone. Frank suffered
from 'fainting spells' that had been diagnosed as epilepsy.

Despite their dissimilarities, perhaps because of them, there was
a wonderful accord between Charles and Frank. Early each morning they set off together to walk to the brewery, which was at the
north end of the town. Alfred said of them, 'Their hats know their

own pegs, so little do these brothers jostle each other in their duties.'
When their work was finished in the afternoon, they left the office
together:

> Charles's arm is through Frank's, and Frank's hand is on the
> hind pocket of his frock-coat. Frank runs off a step or two to
> deposit the money, after which the chances are they take a turn
> through the Market Row; it is full, if it is Market Day; both
> Charles and Frank are sociable, and observant in such a crowd.
> If some birthday be near, they are obliged to make up their
> minds what to purchase for their sister out of the small choice
> in the windows. But the dinner hour is near, and home come the
> last of those, whose labours have earned the meat that is put
> upon the table. Ring the bell, and do not talk to hungry men till
> the first dish is removed!

> Both the Brothers and their father must again go down to the
> brewery in the evening. To Charles the pang of leaving behind
> all his pleasant leisure employments is great enough to cause a
> murmur; he makes others feel that he must go against his will.
> But Frank's disappearance is without a word of notice; indeed
> one might fancy him still busy about the house, so unseen is the
> moment and set of his departure. As for their father, he follows
> regularly, as if it were not form and for countenance sake only.
> He gets health by the walk to the North End, and will do it on a
> Sunday even, when the Office doors are of course closed against
> him as against others. He will strike with his stick on the post
> at the North End, I believed, till the day of his death.[14]

Samuel Paget shouldered not only his own family's problems,
but also those of widowed sisters and cousins. From his dwindling
resources he strove to meet an endless succession of bills. Whenever a special effort was needed to raise a sum of money for one
member of the family, the others were all made to feel that it was
a privilege to be able to help. Thus adversity strengthened family
loyalty. But there were still happy occasions to be enjoyed. Family
celebrations of birthdays and St Valentine's Day continued, despite
Arthur's absence. Mrs Paget, helped by Patty and Kate, still baked
a prodigious array of cakes and sweetmeats; gifts, though fewer,
simpler, and more ingeniously contrived, were still exchanged and
the house often rang with laughter, as it had in the past.

Such was the family life that James knew so well and from which
he was soon to be separated. By mid-1834 he was preparing to go
to London for the next phase of his medical training. In later life he
was able to assess the merits of the apprenticeship system, which
by then had been abandoned:

I cannot doubt that the period thus spent was too long. The first year of it might have been more usefully spent in some good school, the last in a London hospital: but the advantages of an apprenticeship were, or at least might be, far greater than is now commonly supposed. Many things of great utility in after-life could be thoroughly learned, things of which the ignorance is now a frequent hindrance to success: such as dispensing, and a practical knowledge of medicines, and the modes of making them; account-keeping; the business-like habits needed for practice; care and neatness and cleanliness in all minor surgery. Besides, in most cases, as in my own, the elements of anatomy could be slowly learned; there was time for reading and for natural history or any branch of science by which the habit of observing might be gained; and there was ample opportunity for observation in practice, without being confused in a crowd of cases in which it is, for a student, equally difficult either to study the whole or to make a good choice. . . .

Thus, after my four and a half years of apprenticeship, and when I was nearly 21, I was to begin my hospital-work with about as much knowledge of anatomy and physiology as, I suppose, an average student of the present time has at the end of his first year's hospital-study; with more knowledge of medicine and surgery than such an one would now have after two or even three years' study; and with an unusual disposition for scientific pursuits, and an unusually educated power of observing.[15]

Chapter 3

The Student in London

When James Paget climbed on to the London-bound coach in October, 1834, he may well have felt that he was reliving a family legend. Forty years previously his father had made the same journey, also in the belief that the capital held the key to his future. But James's sojourn there would be longer; he now planned to spend two winter terms as a student at a London hospital.

Apprenticeship to a general practitioner had absorbed only a fraction of his capacity to work; his exuberant mental energy had spilled over into the study of other branches of science and the co-authorship of the book on natural history. In London he would be able to concentrate on training for his profession. His teachers would be some of the leading men of the medical world, and he would have much better opportunities for learning than he had had in Yarmouth. As a member of a larger student body he would also be better able to measure his progress against that of his contemporaries.

James joins George at St Bartholomew's Hospital

The hospital he selected was St Bartholomew's. This had been the medical school of Charles Costerton and also of his cousin, Dr Henry Moor. But a more important reason for his choice was that St Bartholomew's was favoured by Cambridge men, and George Paget was already there. George had been awarded the MB, Cambridge in 1833, and was now receiving his clinical training. For a few months the brothers would be able to share lodgings and help each other with their studies.

The oldest London hospital

St Bartholomew's is the oldest of the great London hospitals.* It was founded in 1123 by a monk named Rahere. As a young man in holy orders Rahere was less interested in spiritual matters than in the wordly pleasures and intrigue at the court of Henry I. Then he experienced a profound change of heart and, as an act of penance, he set out on a pilgrimage to Rome. During the journey he contracted malaria and came close to death. Rahere vowed that, if he survived, he would found a refuge for London's sick and destitute. Saint Bartholomew appeared to him in a vision, instructing him to

---

*St Thomas's Hospital also dates from the twelfth century, but it began more tentatively and there is no reliable documentation of its foundation.

build his house of charity at Smithfield, on swampy land that had once been a place of execution. Rahere recovered his health and made his way back to London. He was faithful to his vow. The Smithfield site, when drained, proved to be so well suited to his purpose that the modern Hospital of St Bartholomew stands on the site of Rahere's original shelter for the poor.

The first Hospital consisted of clusters of buildings surrounding several small courtyards. This design provided a sheltered environment for those inmates who were not bedridden, and also helped to foster a community feeling. Close by there was a priory for the Austin Canons who, with the help of a small group of nuns, conducted the institution. In addition to tending the sick, they cared for orphans and sheltered the homeless. But in succeeding centuries, as the treatment of disease became more specialized, the Hospital gave up its other functions. St Bartholomew's Hospital came to play an important role in the life of the city of London. Rich benefactors supported it with gifts of money and property, and the income from its properties enabled it to continue to treat the sick poor without charge.

When the monasteries were dissolved in the reign of Henry VIII the priory was closed, but the Hospital survived. Its management was placed in secular hands and the staff who cared for the patients henceforth were also lay men and women. However, the women who nursed the sick continued to be known as 'Sisters', as the nuns before them had been.

Henry VIII gave the Hospital a royal charter. He appointed a board of governors consisting of four aldermen and eight councillors of the City of London and directed that the City should make an annual contribution to the upkeep of the Hospital. He also tried to change its name to 'The House of the Poor in West Smithfield', but the people of London much preferred the old name, so this edict of the King was ignored.

Other institutions were more harshly treated. In 1540 St Thomas's Hospital, which had been caring for the sick poor of London for four hundred years, was forced to close. The house of St Mary of Bethlehem, or Bethlem, as it came to be known, sheltered the sick and mentally deranged; it was deprived of so much of its income that it was barely able to continue.

Growing public concern at the plight of the poor, and fears of epidemics of the plague, prompted influential citizens to take steps to remedy the situation. During the reign of Edward VI the Corporation of the City of London imposed taxes on the guilds and companies of the prosperous craftsmen and merchants, to help meet the cost of caring for the needy. St Thomas's Hospital was re-opened in 1552. In the same year the Lord Mayor, Sir Richard Dobbes, appealed to the rich to contribute directly. The money so raised was used to support St Bartholomew's, St Thomas's, and Bethlem, and also to establish Christ's Hospital, a home where orphaned boys could receive some education and be trained for useful occupations. An appeal to the King by Bishop Nicholas Ridley resulted in the palace of Bridewell being granted to the City for use as an institution for the housing and occupational training of vagrants.

Thus, by the end of the reign of Edward VI there were in London five institutions, the 'Royal Hospitals', which were supported and governed by the Corporation of the City of London. They are all still in existance, although only St Bartholomew's occupies its original site. Two of them have become schools; Christ's Hospital, relocated to Horsham in Sussex, is the famous Blue-coat School, while Bridewell is now King Edward's School in Witley, Surrey. The schools have retained their association with the City of London, but the hospitals—St Bartholomew's, St Thomas's, and Bethlem—have been incorporated in the National Health Service.

A notable event in the history of St Bartholomew's Hospital was the publication, in 1628, of William Harvey's book *On the Motion of the Heart and Blood in Animals.* Harvey, who was appointed physician to the Hospital in 1609, had doubted even as a student the truth of the then current theory of the function of the heart. It was thought that the blood oscillated, rather than flowing as a stream with a constant direction, and that the arteries contained air as well as blood. By a series of animal experiments Harvey established that two separate streams of blood flow through the heart, one being directed to the lungs, the other to the remainder of the body. He showed that the blood did not oscillate in the blood vessels, but moved in one direction only; he proved that the blood vessels contained only blood and not air. Harvey's discoveries were of the utmost importance. Not only had he elucidated the function of the heart, but he had introduced into medicine the scientific method of discovery by direct observation and experiment.

The Hospital survived several crises in the seventeenth century. It continued to function during the Civil War, although there were conflicts in loyalty between members of the staff and also among the patients. Harvey, who was the King's physician, was forced to resign from the Hospital in 1643. He remained in retirement until his death in 1657. During the outbreak of plague in 1665 many of the staff, including the two physicians, joined the exodus from the city, but the matron, Margaret Blague, bravely remained at her post. Later in the same year the Great Fire burned right up to the Hospital's boundaries. Although the main buildings were unscathed some of the adjacent shops and houses belonging to the Hospital were destroyed. The loss of rental income from these was the more severely felt because, for some years, the City of London had failed to pay its annual contribution to the Hospital. Five of the fifteen wards had to be closed temporarily.

Nevertheless, by the end of the century the Governors were able to begin planning the restoration of some of the buildings that had fallen into disrepair. The north gate leading into Smithfield was rebuilt. The man responsible for its design and construction was the stonemason Edward Strong. Strong's classic design is dominated by a statue of Henry VIII, whose familiar figure gives a human warmth to the appearance of the hospital entrance.

In 1710 the City was compelled by law to pay its debts to the Hospital and there were also a number of generous benefactions. With their new wealth the Governors were able to embark on an

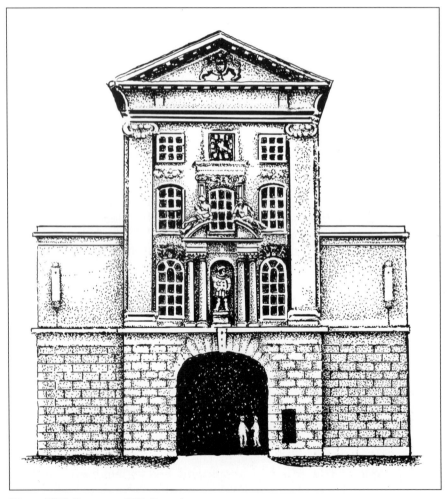

Henry VIII Gateway. (HP Orson).

ambitious rebuilding programme. The architect responsible for the grand design was James Gibbs, who already had to his credit the church of St Martin-in-the-Fields. Gibbs hoped that the new Hospital would not only be suited to its function, but would also be a source of visual pleasure to the people of London. Retaining the original courtyard design, he planned four wings, each of three storeys, surrounding a large rectangular space. At each corner of the quadrangle a gateway provided communication with the adjacent streets. The Henry VIII Gate would lead into the quadrangle via a shallow forecourt that would provide additional insulation from the bustle of Smithfield.

The first of the four main buildings to be completed was the North Wing. The fourth, the East Wing, was not completed until 1769. Financial constraints and shortages of some of the building materials made compromises necessary, and there were still the adjacent rows of shabby properties to mar the visual effect.

This mixture of grandeur and shabbiness impressed Paget when he first glimpsed the Hospital in October, 1834. Fifty years later, when addressing students at St Bartholomew's, he recalled the Hospital as it had been in his own student days:

The hospital itself had all its chief features nearly as you see them now. The square was, in some things, rather more picturesque, for the stone used in all the wings was soft and was, in

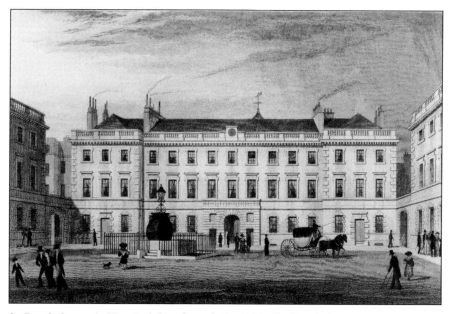

St Bartholomew's Hospital Quadrangle in 1830. (St Bartholomew's Hospital).

many places, worn and flaking; so that the walls had a more ancient look than they have had since they were faced with the smooth hard stone that now covers them. The square looked more like a quad in one of the older Oxford colleges. Besides, at the four corners the wings were connected by well proportioned gateways, and over one of these, at the corner next to the present operating theatre and the adjoining wards, and on the ground now occupied by them, one saw the trees of a garden around what was then the Treasurer's house. It was a fair-sized garden shading a good house, and with fruit trees, and adjoined the garden of the vicarage, which was then close by the church. The good old vicar, Mr Wix, at whose death many years ago the vicarage was pulled down, was proud of his fruit, and especially of the mulberries, which he could gather every year. London-city was then by some miles nearer to the open country, and thirty years earlier there were signs of its being nearer still; for I heard from Dr Hue, who was senior physician when I came to the school, and whose pupilage must have been at the very beginning of this century, that nightingales used to sing in that garden. They were the contemporaries of the historic snipes in the site of Belgravia.

But, if we seem to have suffered loss in these things, we have gained more in others. Where the college and the house-surgeons' rooms now are there was a long row of dirty and often noisy backs of houses, and between these and the east wing, or the new wing as it was then called, there was a shabby line of little two-storied houses in which box-carriers and other hospital-servants lived, and let lodgings to students who wished to be near their work. Worse than this, in the square itself, where now the fountain stands, there was an extremely ugly pump and neither tree nor flower; and, worse still, the square was at that time a thoroughfare all day for foot-passengers. It had none of the quietness in which you can talk and lounge, and in which convalescents can sit and lie about on couches; it was traversed, in the line between Little Britain and Giltspur Street, by any number of people, including, on Mondays and Fridays, which were the Smithfield market-days, many drovers with their sheep-dogs, and, on all days but Saturdays, many poor old clothes-men, who were bullied with the sort of Judenhasse which was not then deemed disgraceful.[1]

James and his brother George shared longings at 9, Charlotte Street during James's first three months in London. George introduced James into the circle of Oxford and Cambridge men, who considered themselves the student elite. James observed, however, that this belief in their superiority beguiled many of these pleasant young gentlemen into a life of idleness, and resulted in their downfall. The canny James 'began at once to work steadily, though often pretending to be rather idle.'

The students were left very much to their own devices. They registered for attendance at lectures but had almost no guidance or supervision. Many students attended lectures at more than one hospital and had no formal attachment to any one institution. Outside the hospital system there were a number of schools offering lectures and demonstrations by noted teachers. These 'grinding schools' competed with the hospitals for fee-paying students. The Aldersgate Street School, which was close to St Bartholomew's Hospital, was one of the most successful.

The medical school was founded by John Abernethy

The medical school at St Bartholomew's began in the seventeenth century, when 'young doctors' in small numbers accompanied senior physicians and surgeons during their visits to the Hospital. As their numbers grew some administrators complained that the students were a nuisance and should be discouraged. The far-sighted, who could see an important role for hospitals as institutions for medical training, were more helpful. Thus a museum for anatomical and surgical specimens was established in 1726. In 1767 the House Committee granted the physicians and surgeons permission to use the operating theatre and an adjoining room as lecture theatres. The famous surgeon Percivall Pott was one of the first to make use of this facility. The medical school was founded by another surgeon, John Abernethy, who was appointed to an assistant post at the Hospital in 1787. Abernethy was not a particularly skilful operator, but he was an excellent lecturer. His ability to impart important principles succinctly and in a memorable fashion ensured that his classes were always crowded. Abernethy lectured on anatomy, physiology, and surgery. Other members of the staff contributed lectures on physic, midwifery, and chemistry, so enabling the Hospital to offer students a complete course of training. The presence of an increasing number of enthusiastic students added to the prestige of the Hospital and stimulated the staff to greater effort. The House Committee consequently accepted Abernethy's proposal that a new lecture theatre should be built. Over four hundred people attended Abernethy's first lecture in the new theatre on 1 October, 1822.

After Abernethy's retirement in 1827 the medical school at St Bartholomew's declined because none of the members of the staff were as devoted to it as he had been. Some of them were excellent teachers, but they were all unable or unwilling to take on his role as advocate for the school and to battle with the Hospital Governors

for improved facilities for students. Consequently, when James
Paget arrived in 1834 enrolments at St Bartholomew's were declin-
ing, while the new University College and the Aldersgate Street
School were flourishing.

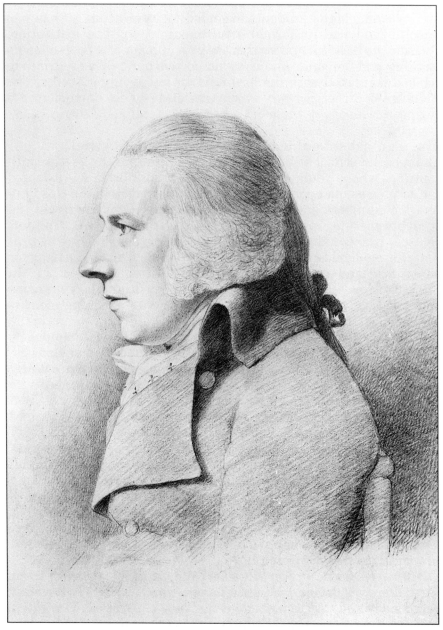

John Abernethy by G Dance, 1793. (National Portrait Gallery).

Paget observed that the name of Abernethy was still greatly revered. The students had named their organisation the Abernethian Society in his honour; his influence was still to be felt throughout the Hospital. Yet Paget, who was inclined to be a hero-worshipper, had his reservations about John Abernethy: '. . . There were some at the Hospital who might have been much stronger men if they had not thought it enough to be like Abernethy, and like enough to him if they imitated his manners . . .' Paget was here referring to Abernethy's reputation for speaking roughly, not only to colleagues but also to his patients; the young Paget found this inexcusable. But among the senior men at the Hospital there were several who won his whole-hearted admiration. His appreciation of two of them is as revealing of Paget himself as it is of Lawrence and Stanley.

(The lectures) of Lawrence were, I think, the best then given in London: admirable in their well collected knowledge, and even more admirable in their order, their perfect clearness of language, and the quietly attractive manner in which they were delivered. As I remember them now, I feel that I did not esteem them half enough at the time. It was a great pleasure to hear them, and a good lesson. They were given on three days in the week at 7 in the evening, after dinner. He used to come to the Hospital in the omnibus, and, after a few minutes in the Museum, would, as the clock struck, enter the theatre, then always full. He came with a strange vague outlook as if with uncertain sight; the expression of his eyes was always inferior to that of his other features. These were impressive, beautiful and grand— significant of vast mental power well trained and well sustained. He came in quietly, and after sitting for about half a minute, as if gathering his thoughts, began, in a clear rather high note, speaking quite deliberately in faultless words as if telling judiciously that which he was just now thinking. There was no hurry, no delay, no repetition, no revision: every word had been learned by heart, and yet there was not the least sign that one word was being remembered. It was the best method of scientific speaking that I have ever heard; and there was no one, at that time, in England, if I may not say in Europe, who had more completely studied the whole principles and practice of Surgery.

Stanley lectured on Anatomy and Physiology every day, Saturdays excepted, at half-past two. The physiological portion of the lectures was, even for that time, feeble; he had never studied chemistry, physics, or any adjacent part of the science, and the physiology of even that time was beyond his grasp. And the anatomy was very elementary: but he lectured so carefully and clearly, he was so deliberate and simple, so grave and earnest, and he repeated all the 'tips' so frequently, without changing one important word, that I believe there was not in London a more instructive teacher than he was. Besides, his occasional attempts at 'style' were so funny that they were easily remembered, easily imitated; and, in association with them, the words he used were well remembered too. It was believed that one of my friends, who afterwards became a distinguished comic writer, passed the College solely by means of the bits of lectures with which he used to make fun by imitating Stanley.

It would be hard to find two men more unlike than were Lawrence and Stanley; and yet it would be hard to say which was the better teacher, if one would reckon the effect not only of their words (for Lawrence's were nearly all in print) but of their personal influence on students. Lawrence was almost inimitable, unless by those of unusual ability and rare cultivation; and he never seemed in difficulty. Stanley made all feel the value of dull hard work, the use of accuracy in common things, the need of learning the very commonest facts: his honest plodding day's work was a lesson to any one who would watch it kindly, and the story of his life was full of teaching. As a boy he was poor and poorly educated; as a hospital-student he was ridiculed and bullied; as a teacher he was opposed, hindered, laughed-at in journals and caricatures; some of his colleagues did their best to make him miserable: and yet he became constantly more esteemed, more trusted, more gladly worked-with by those who knew him well; and these became constantly more numerous; for he was completely honest, true and truth-loving, keenly conscious of his duty and resolute in doing it.

It was singularly happy for me that I had the teaching and the example of both Lawrence and Stanley: I learned nothing but what was good from either of them and, even in the later intimacy of colleagueship and friendship into which I grew, found constantly more to esteem in both, even though the contrast between their intellectual characters became more marked.[2]

James plans to be a surgeon
Paget's apprenticeship had been intended to prepare him for general practice, but it seems that even before he arrived at the surgically orientated Hospital he had already decided to devote himself solely to the study of surgery. Preparation for the examination of the Society of Apothecaries formed no part of his plan of study. Lack of this qualification would not necessarily debar him from general practice, but his ambitions were beginning to take a different direction.

He found that, apart from the lectures, there was very little formal teaching at the Hospital. An able and industrious student could readily acquire there all the knowledge he needed to pass the examinations, but he had to devise his own curriculum. James spent each morning in the dissecting room, working with the aid of Stanley's *Anatomy* and the *Dublin Dissector*. His afternoons and evenings were spent in studying, interspersed with lectures and post-mortem demonstrations. He read avidly from the standard text-books and journals—Turner's *Chemistry*, Mayo's *Physiology*, the *Lancet* and the *Cyclopaedia of Medicine*. He translated more French text-books to add to his collection. The most important of these was Cloquet's *Anatomy*, which he found invaluable. His friends observed with amusement that his Cloquet manuscript was the first of his possessions that he thought of saving when there was a fire in the house next door to his lodgings.

He was advised to learn German as well, since much of the best work in anatomy and physiology was then being published by German scientists. He quickly acquired a working knowledge of this language and produced his own translation of Hildebrandt's *Anatomie* and Muller's articles on the physiology of the liver and the nervous system. He was delighted that Stanley included in his lectures some information obtained from student Paget's German translations. Seldom, he thought, had a student attracted the favourable attention of a lecturer by so simple a means.

A frugal and studious life in London

James Paget's first term in London set the pattern of his life for many years to come. It was a frugal existence. Even the smallest expenditure had to be carefully considered and there was nothing to spare for theatres, restaurants, or sight-seeing. Fortunately, he found his work utterly absorbing and was happy to spend most evenings working late over his books. When his brother George left London just after Christmas James must have occasionally yearned to be back in the house on the Quay, or wandering in the Norfolk countryside, as he had when gathering his plant specimens. But it seems that neither homesickness nor loneliness ever presented any serious problem. Friendships, both new and old, helped him to adjust to isolation from his family.

Among his fellow students there were a number who were congenial company and who became life-long friends. He also enjoyed the hospitality of the Revd Henry North and family. Two of Mr North's sons had been curates at Yarmouth, where they became friendly with the Pagets. In London James was made welcome at the North home and was glad to spend many of his Sunday evenings there, enjoying conversation and music-making. He maintained the Paget tradition of letter-writing. A constant stream of letters passed between London and the house on the Quay. George and James also kept each other fully informed about the progress of their studies and exchanged news of mutual friends.

Not all of James's fellow students were able to order their lives so satisfactorily. Some were doubtless unsuited to their chosen vocation and were bound to fail. Others could perhaps have succeeded if they had been guided and disciplined but, left to their own devices, they drifted into idleness. The poor facilities for students were partly to blame. Although the Hospital had a medical library, from which books could be borrowed, there was no reading room. The students clubbed together to rent a room over a baker's shop near the Hospital. Here they could read journals and study in the intervals between lectures. Many of them formed the habit of spending their evenings there as well, playing cards and talking, rather than returning to their cheerless lodgings to study. Others were led further astray and, having succumbed to drinking and gambling, disappeared from the ranks of the students.

Contemporary student behaviour
Medical students of the first half of the nineteenth century have a reputation for profligacy. Viewed in retrospect from the decorous later Victorian era, they appeared devoid of any admirable qualities. Unwashed, immoral, coarse in speech and behaviour, they apparently lacked all the qualities that a patient would seek in his medical adviser. Paget certainly encountered some who fitted this description but when, as an old man, he recalled his fellow students he thought that their failings were a reflection of the times in which they lived:

> As for the general body of the students of my time, I believe they were, in comparison with others of the same age and same level, about as they are now. I cannot venture to say whether they were a little better or a little worse than young lawyers or young men of business. As among other students, there were a few thoroughly vicious fellows who came to a bad end, left the school in disgrace, or were plucked and not heard of more; and some idle fools, and some blockheads and untaught, who could never learn their duty. These have been caricatured as if they were types of the whole class; it would be as reasonable to sketch the general characteristics of Englishmen from a slight acquaintance with some inmates of a lunatic asylum. The majority of students then, as now, worked well; some were laborious, as with a natural pleasure in the exercise of mental power, or in emulation, or in consciousness of duty or of necessity, or with all these motives. Some of these are living still . . . I doubt whether you could find better now.

There is a greater contrast in the play than in the work of that time and this. The pleasures and amusements then were coarser. There was much more drinking; a few were often drunk, and many who never were so would boast of drinking more than they thought they needed. Cursing and swearing were common in ordinary talk, frequent for emphasis, and nasty stories were very often told and deemed of the same worth as witty ones. Impurity of life and conversation were scarcely thought disgraceful or worth concealing. But in all these faults there were great differences among the students; some might boast of them, but many only tolerated them and kept as clear as they could; a few rebuked them, chiefly those who, in the slang of those days, were called Saints or Simeonites, after the great Cambridge preacher. But let me repeat, the students of that time were only living and talking after the ordinary manner of the day; the same faults, the same virtues, prevailed in all similar groups of men, just as now you who are temperate and pure and decent in your language are not rare examples of the men of these much better times in which you live.[3]

Some of the teachers were severely censured by their contemporaries for their use of bad language and indecent stories in their lectures to students. The culprits argued that bawdy jokes and mnemonics helped the students to remember otherwise dull facts. It was even argued by some that the need to use such aids to memory was a reason why women could never be admitted as medical students. Paget was so disgusted by the teachers of midwifery that he attended only two lectures on the subject. He described their language as 'pitch from the defilement of which one feels even now not quite cleansed.'

Hard work rewarded
Early in 1835, after George Paget had returned to Cambridge, James moved to new lodgings at 12, Thavies Inn. He shared these with his friend Johnstone, who was his senior by several years. Johnstone, an able young physician, was highly regarded by his seniors at the Hospital. In 1834 the students at St Bartholomew's had, for the first time, been invited to enter for competitive examinations. These were so successful that they were held again in 1835. Paget decided to try for the prizes in medicine, surgery, chemistry, and botany. To his astonishment he won all four. He later recalled: 'The surprise was the cause of one of the only two sleepless nights which I have ever had, unless in severe illness.'

Paget discovers *Trichina spiralis*
In the same year he had an even more gratifying success. In

February, 1835, he made an original discovery that attracted considerable attention and resulted in the name of James Paget appearing for the first time in the medical literature. He was the first to observe the parasite *Trichina spiralis* in a human subject. The *Trichina* organism is a minute worm that is found in immature, or larval, form in the muscle tissue of swine. Humans acquire the infestation by eating raw or improperly cooked pork. In the human

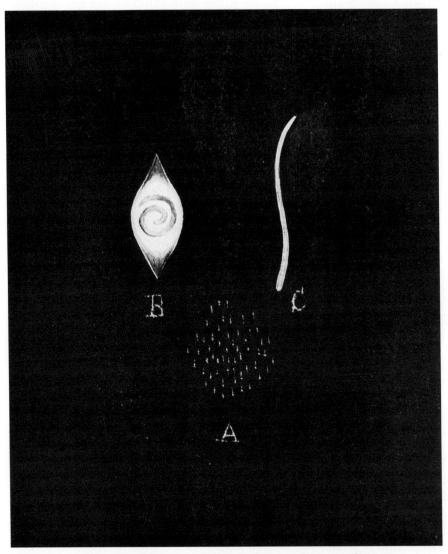

Paget's Drawings of the Trichina parasite. A, Cysts of the natural size as scattered among the muscular fibres; B, Single cyst containing the worm, magnified ; C, Worm removed from the cyst and uncoiled. (Royal College of Surgeons of England).

stomach the larvae become active and, on entering the bowel of the host, they multiply rapidly. In vast numbers they penetrate the wall of the bowel, enter the bloodstream, and are eventually carried to the lungs. From the lungs they are distributed throughout the body, but are found in greatest number in the muscles. Over a period of several weeks thousands of these minute parasites may become lodged in the muscles of the host. The unfortunate victim suffers severe muscular pain, fever, congestion of the lungs, and pneumonia. Death may occur at this stage, but in milder cases the symptoms gradually subside. The parasites in the muscles eventually die and each becomes encased, or encysted, in a calcific shell, so that it later appears as a gritty particle.

When Paget made his discovery the disease was widespread in Europe, but its nature was not recognized; nobody had attached any significance to the minute sand-like granules that were frequently found at post-mortem examinations. One may well wonder how it was that a student who had been at the Hospital for less than six months was able to discover something that had been overlooked by more experienced men. Paget's description of the attitude to post-mortem examinations at the Hospital provides an explanation:

> The dead-house (it was never called by any better name) was a miserable kind of shed, stone-floored, damp, and dirty, where all stood round a table on which the examinations were made. And these were usually made in the roughest and least instructive way; and, unless one of the physicians were present, nothing was carefully looked-at, nothing was taught. Pathology, in any fair sense of the word, was hardly considered.[4]

If missed at the post-mortem examination, the condition was equally likely to escape the attention of the Curator of the museum.

> The Curator was Mr Bayntin, a very neat and careful dissector, a clever pretty artist, admirable in all the mechanical part of his work, but, whether through idleness or weakly health, not studious, not ready to go beyond that part of it; his study of anatomy, whether normal or morbid, was completed when an illustration of it, well dissected, was displayed in clear colourless spirit, in a well-fitted bottle, air-tight, with a perfectly well-painted cover, duly numbered and very briefly catalogued.[5]

Paget believed that it was his training as a botanist that had enabled him to make the discovery:

> All the men in the dissecting-rooms, teachers included, 'saw' the little specks in the muscles: but I believed that I alone 'looked-at'

them and 'observed' them: no one trained in natural history could have failed to do so.[6]

The patient in whom Paget's observations were made was a middle-aged Italian named Paolo Bianchi. Bianchi's death had been caused by tuberculosis, a disease not then recognized as a bacterial infection. The gritty specks in his muscles had not directly contributed to his death. Paget took specimens of muscle for microscopic examination but, as St Bartholomew's Hospital did not have a microscope, he sought the help of some of his distinguished botanist friends and was given a letter of introduction to Robert Brown of the British Museum. At the Hospital Paget found himself competing with one of his teachers, Dr Richard Owen, the lecturer in comparative anatomy. He wrote of these events in a letter to his brother Charles:

> You will I think be interested in hearing that I have lately discovered a perfectly new animalcule, infesting in myriads the human muscles during life—little worms about 1/30 of an inch long coiled up in minute cells as you see in the drawing which I have sent with this. I made out clearly their intestines and have measured all their dimensions and the account is to be published either in the Transactions of the Zoological or of the Medico-Chirurgical Society. I do not yet know whether I shall write the description myself, or whether Mr Owen our lecturer on Comparative Anatomy will do it. I should rather think the latter, as he having used far more powerful microscopes than I had, has been able to make out their organisation more clearly. Whichever be the case, I have taken care that I should receive at least some credit for the discovery, though this was not to be had without some trouble.

> Their occurrence is by no means uncommon having been observed in several cases in the dissecting rooms, but overlooked or mistaken for little bits of bone. The fact of this occurrence is itself interesting and from their immense number may prove important when more cases have been found and compared, so as to see whether they accompany any particular disease. The present was a case of consumption. Fancy the body of a single individual supporting more separately existing creatures than the population of the whole world, and there must in this subject have been 10 times as many. However you shall see the paper as soon as it is published.

> I have already reaped some of the benefits of the discovery in a favourable introduction to Brown—*the* Brown who alone of the

whole world of that name would be known without the adjunct
of some Christian appellation—the best botanist perhaps in the
world. He was remarkably kind and lent me his microscope. Mr
Children too I saw about it and made my peace with him, my not
having called on him before having rather lowered me in his
estimation. I have obtained by it too an introduction to Mr
Longstaff, who has the best anatomical and surgical (private)
museum in England, and he has invited me to see it some day this
week. Mr Kirby too will be up in London soon and he is to see
them. All this looks like making progress in *something* at least
and I hope may in time bring some tangible fruits.[7]

By presenting his findings at a meeting of the Abernethian
Society Paget established his claim to the discovery of the parasite.
He was content to share his success with Owen, who had the honour
of naming the organism. Fortunately, there was no enmity between
Paget and Owen as a result of the *Trichina* episode. Paget later
recalled:

. . . Owen, to whom specimens were taken when I had seen that
there was a 'worm', read a paper on it at the Zoological Society,
and gave it its name. It mattered little: the repute of the
discovery would have been of no great use to me: and I should
have gained less happiness by disputing for it and obtaining it
than I have enjoyed in the personal friendship with Owen ever
since. It was enough for my advantage that the discovery, and
the paper at the Abernethian, strengthened my position in the
Hospital.[8]

History has duly acknowledged the contributions of both men.
Twenty-five years later the German scientists Virchow and von
Zenker completed the story of the life cycle of the parasite.
    In recalling the achievements of his first term in London, Paget
suggests that they were pleasing, but of no great importance:

The consequence of this success on my position in the school was
considerable, and its influence on myself was, I think, harmless.
At the most it may have increased a belief that I might become
connected with the Hospital and be prosperous in London: but it
was not enough to change any plans or anything in the course of
my work.[9]

Yet in this comment he revealed an important change in his
outlook. He was contemplating remaining permanently in London,
practising as a consultant surgeon, with an appointment at St
Bartholomew's Hospital. As an apprentice he had been disap-

pointed to find that much of the work done by men like Charles Costerton had become routine and was probably of little value. In London he had witnessed a much more satisfying professional life. A consultant surgeon in the city could continually extend the range of his knowledge and skills; he could be a scientist, as well as a healer of wounds. Paget was beginning to realize that this dual role was ideally suited to his own temperament.

He returned to Yarmouth between his first and second winter terms at the Hospital. There was very little teaching of any kind during the summer so, like most students whose homes were outside London, he preferred to save the cost of lodgings by remaining at home until the next winter term was about to begin. In October, 1835 he was back at 12, Thavies Inn.

More time in the wards
In their second year of study the students had fewer formal lectures and spent more time in the wards. As an apprentice in Yarmouth Paget had seen poverty and disease, but in the wards of St Bartholomew's Hospital he was to become much more familiar with these twin causes of human suffering. The Hospital that Paget knew was a large institution. Although in 1547 Henry VIII had decreed that it should be limited to one hundred inpatients, this restriction was later removed and the Hospital continued to grow. In 1835 its twenty-eight wards contained over five hundred patients, all of whom were cared for without charge. Nearly all of its patients were very poor, but there were a few exceptions, as the Hospital Commissioners' Report of 1837 noted:

> The majority of those received as patients into the hospital are mechanics, labourers, reduced tradesmen or servants. There are, however, numerous admissions of individuals of both sexes, and particularly females of the very lowest class of society and the worst character. It occasionally happens that, in serious cases of casualty, opulent persons are brought to the hospital and admitted as accident patients, but there is no apartment peculiarly appropriated for them, and they are placed in the ordinary wards indiscriminately with the poor patients.[10]

As soon as they were well enough to be moved the 'opulent persons' would have returned to their homes. At that time nobody who could be cared for at home chose to be in hospital, no matter how grave his illness. Even serious operations were performed in private residences.

The only persons debarred from admission to St Bartholomew's were those thought to be suffering from smallpox. Accident victims and sick people found lying in the streets were brought to the Hospital at any time of day or night, and were never turned away. The Hospital had once employed its own beadles to go out looking for these unfortunates, but after the formation of the police force in 1829 this work ceased to be the responsibility of Hospital servants.

St Bartholomew's wards were of two sizes: 'double' wards with about thirty beds, and 'single' wards with half that number. A ward was a little community whose inmates shared the joy of a recovery from desperate illness or the tragedy of a death. Each bed was fitted with curtains of plain blue or checked fabric that could be drawn to give the occupant some small measure of privacy. Convalescent patients sometimes helped the nurses, but others became quite unruly as they regained their health and strength. Such offences as smoking, swearing, gambling and fighting could result in a patient's being summarily discharged and treated as an outpatient.

Paget observed that the wards were scrupulously clean, but nobody then knew that even the highest domestic standards were not sufficient for hospitals. Seemingly clean hands and equipment were the unsuspected carriers of infection from one patient to another. One unusual amenity that the Hospital enjoyed was a piped water supply to all the wards. Most householders in the neighbourhood had to carry their water by the bucketful from the local pump. Warm baths were another luxury. The Hospital Commissioners' Report notes:

> As soon as the patients have been examined by the principal physician or surgeon, such of them as are admitted and require it are washed in the warm bath, of which there is one fixed on every floor except the upper floor, and are then put to bed.[11]

Nevertheless, frequent bathing thereafter could not have been encouraged, since the bath was usually covered with a large board on which plates were laid when the patients' meals were being dished up!

Candles lit the wards at night. Although gaslight brightened the streets of London, it was not in general use for interior lighting. Even the House of Commons was still candle-lit, although there the candles were mounted in elaborate chandeliers. The wards of St Bartholomew's in general compared favourably with those of other London hospitals. Paget recalled:

> The interiors of the wings were not very different from what they are now, except that all three were, as the west wing has become since the clearing-away of the nurses' rooms. They all had, as that has now, the admirable wide open air space between the wards and the unhindered access to the broad staircase; a plan

unmatched in any hospital that I have ever seen. And the wards were as they are now in size and shape and airiness; but were bare of all look of gladness or decoration; not a picture, not a flower, not a text, not one look of brightness or of cheer was in them. Very gloomy and sad you may say, but it was consistent with all that was without. Not a church had then a decoration; London was almost without flowers; there were no popular graphic arts, no cheap good arts of any kind; so there was no distress of contrast, and it is in contrasts, I suppose, that are the chief of all our pleasures and pains.[12]

Most of the patients probably thought the wards quite pleasing, since many had been homeless and hungry, as well as sick, when they came to the Hospital for help. Frequently the clothing they arrived in was fit only to be burned. The Hospital maintained a stock from which the needy could be outfitted when they were ready to be discharged. Efforts were also made to find them employment and somewhere to live.

The most valuable service the Hospital provided for some patients was to give them nourishment, and rest in clean beds. The diet, for those who were not restricted because they were suffering from fever, was ample but monotonous. The daily ration consisted of a serving of milk porridge, 12 oz. of bread, 6 oz. of mutton or beef, and 1 pint of broth with peas or potatoes; male patients were each allowed 2 pints of beer, females 1 pint. The beer, which was brewed at the Hospital, was probably of low alcohol content. Tea and sugar were not included in the standard diet, but were available if requested. Butter (1 oz.) was served only on Tuesdays and Fridays. A 'scurvy drink' prepared by the Sisters helped to prevent the vitamin deficiencies that would otherwise have resulted from a diet so lacking in fruit and vegetables.

Nursing staff overworked but kindly
The wards at St Bartholomew's bore biblical names or the names of men associated with the history of the Hospital. The same name was adopted by the Sister in charge of the ward. Thus Paget tells of the loyal service given by Sister Hope and Sister Rahere. The custom was continued in later years when special wards were added to the Hospital; the ranks of the Sisters thus came to include Sister Casualty and even Sister Eyes! Paget described the Sisters and nurses he had known in his student days:

> . . . There were some excellent nurses, especially among the sisters in the medical wards, where everything was more gentle and more orderly than in the surgical. There was an admirable Sister Hope, who had had her leg amputated in the hospital and then

spent her life in giving others the most kindly watchful care. A
Sister Mary, a near relative of hers, was as constant to her
charge; and there were some good surgical sisters too. They had
none of the modern art; they could not have kept a chart or
skilfully taken a temperature, but they had an admirable sagac-
ity and a sort of rough practical knowledge which were nearly as
good as any acquired skill. An old Sister Rahere was the chief
among them, stout, ruddy, positive, very watchful. She once
taught an erring house-surgeon where and how to compress a
posterior tibial artery; she could always report correctly the
progress of a case; and from her wages she saved all she could and
left it in legacy to the hospital. And there was her neighbour,
Sister Colston, rough-tongued, scolding, not seldom rather tipsy;
and yet very watchful and really very helpful, especially in what
she felt to be good cases. On the whole, indeed, it may fairly be
said that the sisters were among the very best nurses of that
time. The ordinary nurses were not so; the greater part of them
were rough, dull, unobservant, and untaught women; of the best
it could only be said that they were kindly, and careful and
attentive in doing what they were told to do.[13]

It is remarkable that any of the nurses were kindly and careful
since, by modern standards, they were all cruelly overworked.

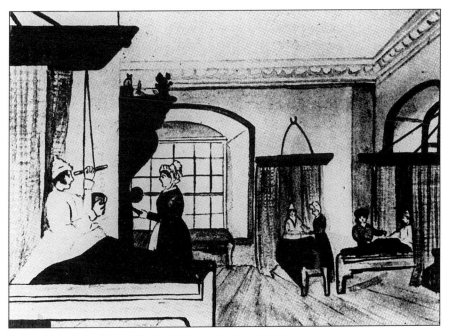

Rahere Ward in 1832. (St Bartholomew's Hospital).

Double wards were staffed by a Sister and three nurses, single wards by a Sister and two nurses. In addition to washing and feeding the patients and keeping their beds neatly made, the nurses had to do the work of charwomen. They swept and scrubbed the floors and kept the furniture and other equipment clean. There was only one unpleasant task they were spared; the Hospital employed a man whose job it was to keep the wooden beds free from the ubiquitous bed-bug. A nurse's working day was fourteen or fifteen hours long and time off duty was granted as a privilege rather than a right. It rarely amounted to more than three or four hours per week. A nurse who felt the need of an occasional tipple could hardly be blamed.

No scientific basis for most treatment
In 1835 biological science was on the threshold of a period of remarkable progress. Developments in the new fields of physiology, biochemistry, microbiology, and pathology were about to transform the practice of medicine. Physicians would not be content to ameliorate the symptoms of disease; they would aim for precise diagnosis, followed by treatment that would remove the cause of the symptoms. But when Paget began his studies in the medical wards most of the forms of treatment he saw in use were time-honoured remedies, for which there was no scientific basis. Thus bleeding, purging, and 'lowering diets' were used for a wide variety of diseases. Another popular remedy was mercury. It was prescribed not only for syphilis but, as Paget noted, for many other undiagnosed chronic inflammations. The side-effects of this treatment were unpleasant:

> It was generally given so as to produce salivation; it was commonly thought not likely to be useful, unless it 'touched the gums'; and, commonly, the syphilitic wards stank foully from the mouths of the patients who were spitting profusely, with swollen gums, and lips and tongues; a hideous sight and stench.[14]

Surgery before anaesthetics and antiseptics
The surgical wards, in the days before antisepsis, also presented a forbidding prospect. Surgery was limited to the treatment of fractures, amputation of severely injured or diseased limbs, drainage of abscesses, and removal of superficial cysts and tumours. Some surgeons specialised in the removal of stones from the bladder. Operations were so frequently followed by overwhelming infection that they were performed only as a desperate measure. Elective surgery, that is surgery undertaken purely to improve the well-being of a patient, was almost unknown. Abdominal operations were so likely to have a fatal outcome that they were rarely

attempted. Bleeding was frequently used as a preliminary to short surgical procedures, in order to reduce the patient to a state of semi-consciousness and muscular relaxation. Paget describes the reduction of a dislocation of the shoulder by this method:

> The patient was set upright on a chair; his arm tied above the elbow and blood let flow from a very free opening in a vein below the tape. So it flowed on and on; and its quantity was hardly measured; it had to be enough to make him faint; and at last he would begin to look pale, and his head would droop and his forehead sweat; and then he would sink down, and slide in his chair, and be hardly conscious and wholly unable to resist the force with which his dislocated limb was pulled at and lifted, and set right. Very horrible, was it not? but what would you do now without the anaesthetics?[15]

Surgeons were proud of their dexterity as operators. Speed was essential, since the patient was conscious, or nearly so, throughout the operation. A thorough knowledge of surgical anatomy and skill in the use of a small range of simple instruments were important elements of this technique. Paget describes one of the acknowledged masters at work:

> I remember it was told, but perhaps not truly, of Sir Astley Cooper, who was a remarkably tall and handsome man, that when an amputation was to be performed, he would enjoy to stand aside, knife in hand, chatting with his friends, while the patient was being placed in due posture and the tourniquet applied. Then, he would step in and, with graceful movements, swiftly remove the limb, tie, perhaps, the one main artery, and then resume his scarcely interrupted conversation while his assistants tied the remaining vessels and dressed the stump.[16]

Despite the brilliance of the surgeon's performance, the wound was certain to become infected. The operator wore his street clothes, the surgical knife had been perfunctorily washed after its last use, and the assistant carried the suture materials in his pocket or threaded through his waistcoat buttonhole. Even if the wound had miraculously escaped infection at the time of operation, it would not remain clean for long. Every surgeon employed a 'box carrier' whose task it was to wash the instruments after an operation and return them to their carrying box. When the surgeon visited his patients in the wards the box carrier walked behind him, handing him the instruments he needed to probe and trim wounds. Instruments used on a hideously infected wound would be wiped on a cloth and returned to the box, ready for use on the next patient.

In Paget's student days the atmosphere of surgical wards was heavy with the odour of discharging wounds. It was little wonder that only the poor were treated in hospitals.

Paget has difficulty in obtaining surgical training

Such, then, were the best and the worst aspects of the wards in which students like Paget sought practical experience. They would accompany a physician or surgeon as he visited his patients, standing with him at the bedside as he demonstrated the special features of each case. This form of teaching is still regarded as invaluable, but it requires that the students be in small groups of not more than half a dozen or so. William Lawrence, the leading surgeon at the Hospital, was held in such high esteem that he attracted crowds of students. Often as many as a hundred tried to follow him around the wards. Most of them could neither hear nor see their teacher; their sole purpose in attending was to be able to claim later that they had been students of the great Lawrence.

The other two surgeons, John Vincent and Henry Earle, were not greatly interested in teaching students. Stanley, whose lectures Paget had found so valuable in his first term, was only an assistant surgeon. This appointment allowed him very few inpatients, so he was not able to give the bedside teaching that the senior students needed. Paget realized that he would have to devise an alternative programme of study that would compensate for this lack of clinical teaching in surgery.

A small number of fortunate students did not have this problem. They were the apprentices of the Hospital surgeons. It was customary for eminent surgeons to accept apprentices, each of whom remained with the same master for four or five years. Unlike the apprentices of general practitioners, these men did not have to perform the menial tasks that Paget knew so well. All of their time was usefully spent in learning their future profession.

The advantages did not end when the student passed his examinations. By long-established custom, appointments to the surgical staff of the Hospital almost invariably went to men who had been apprenticed to Hospital surgeons. Thus, among the students, the apprentices formed an elite group, from which Paget was excluded.

Since worthwhile tuition in surgery seemed to be beyond his reach, Paget decided on a course that was rather unorthodox for a man who was determined to be a surgeon; he would spend most of his time in the medical wards, and would attend the ward rounds of the physician Dr Peter Mere Latham.

Dr Latham's teaching was admirable. With feeble health, and often asthmatic, he used to come down at least three times a week at 8 in the morning; and he would make those who went

round with him examine for themselves, and would tell and
show them how to learn, and have his case-books well kept, and,
in short, follow all the methods which I believe are now used by
the best clinical teachers. This precision, and the early hours,
were too much for the great majority of students: and even
Latham was seldom attended by more than some twelve or
fourteen of the better working men. But of these I think there
were none who did not thoroughly admire him, and imitate him
in his mode of study, and very gratefully remember his teaching.[17]

While benefitting from this excellent teaching in medicine, Paget
had to be careful not to neglect his surgery. He performed as many
post-mortem examinations and dissections as he could, read texts
on anatomy and surgery, and discussed these subjects with his
fellow students. Early in 1836 he had to find new lodgings, probably
because his friend Johnstone was about to enter private practice.
He moved to 82, Hatton Gardens, where his fellow lodgers were
Firth and Master, Norwich men who had become his friends during
the first term. In that term another student had complained that
'Master Jimmy Paget was always sneaking about the dissecting
room at eight o'clock in the morning'. He must have been even more
irritated by Paget's behaviour during this second term, when he
was relying on dissecting to help prepare him for his surgical
examination.

The unusual course of study that Paget followed had an important influence on his later career. His great strengths were the
breadth of his knowledge and his diagnostic ability, qualities that
he probably acquired as a result of this early blending of medical
and surgical training. His exclusion from the practical surgery that
his apprentice colleagues enjoyed in such liberal measure also had
a lasting effect. He was always conscious of this early deficiency in
his training and, although he later took steps to remedy it, he never
claimed to be a brilliant operator.

Further academic success
In his second year Paget again entered for the competitive examinations at the Hospital, and again was outstandingly successful.
He was awarded the first places in Anatomy and Physiology,
Clinical Medicine, and Jurisprudence. The last subject was one
that he had not studied seriously and he had entered for it almost
as an afterthought. He 'crammed' for a few days before the examination in order to obtain a superficial knowledge of the subject. He
was almost ashamed to have won the prize in this way, but in later
life he observed that 'The capacity to "cram" is a most useful power,
essential to the success of many in high station, especially Cabinet
Ministers and leading barristers.'

In May, 1836, he took the Membership examination of the Royal College of Surgeons. There were no written papers. Each candidate appeared before ten examiners who were seated at a long table. Paget had no difficulty with the questions on anatomy; his translations from the French and German anatomists had given him a knowledge of the subject that exceeded the requirements of the examiners. His only anxious moments were when two of them, Mr White and Sir Astley Cooper, questioned him on finer points of surgical technique. At the end of the twenty-minute examination Paget was informed that he had passed. He would be admitted to the Membership of the Royal College of Surgeons.

The joy of achievement was soon mingled with anxiety about his future prospects. If he returned to Yarmouth he could begin to practise immediately and would soon be self-supporting. On the other hand, London held the promise of far greater professional fulfilment and, eventually, better financial rewards. But the immediate future in London was uncertain; it could be years before he was able to establish a practice there.

The problem was as important to his father as it was to James. Samuel Paget had come to London for the Hospital prize-giving, held two days before the college examination. He wrote to Betsey about his dilemma:

> I am just returned from the Hospital with dear James, and I am most amply repaid for my journey if nothing else comes of it. Nothing could exceed the unequivocal testimony from all the physicians, also Mr Laurence, Mr Earle, & Mr Stanley, and, indeed, every one to me *personally* as to his abilities—his industry and his private worth, and I do really believe they would, if they could or can, give him something. Mr Earle, in particular, said something must be found, the Hospital ought not to lose sight of him; and I myself can see plainly it would also be a popular thing as an encouragement to future students to exert themselves. He was immensely cheered, I assure you, on taking his Prizes—the Hall was very full with Ladies, Gentlemen, and Students. It is indeed most gratifying to all of us, and most creditable to him — all my fear is the expense, if he is to follow these schools. Where am I to find the money? for it must be a further great outlay, till they could give him (if they are sincere) something. On the other hand, he must, if he could take the chance and remain here, in time do infinitely better than he could expect to do in the country...[18]

Father and son spent a few days together in London and then returned to Yarmouth. No decision had been made and James's future was to be given more careful consideration over the next few weeks.

Chapter 4

Working, Waiting, and Hoping

It was difficult for James to think objectively about his problems once he rejoined the family at Yarmouth. Alfred, his youngest brother, was now a student at Cambridge, preparing for his entry into the Church. Of the seven brothers who had grown up together, only Charles and Frank remained at home; as the household diminished, its members felt their interdependence even more strongly. James knew that his family would have been pleased to see him settle in Yarmouth as a general practitioner, doing the work he had learned as Charles Costerton's apprentice. But his experience in London had convinced him that this was not his true vocation.

There is an interesting parallel to Paget's dilemma in George Eliot's novel *Middlemarch*. The story traces the career of Tertius Lydgate, an idealistic young surgeon who tried to establish himself in practice in a conservative English village. His advanced scientific ideas and unwillingness to dispense traditional potions earned him the enmity of the older doctors in the neighbourhood and the distrust of potential patients. Lydgate was an unhappy failure. George Eliot is renowned for her accuracy in such matters, so the attitudes she ascribes to Middlemarch in the 1830s probably prevailed in many villages and provincial towns at that time.

As October approached, James was drawn irresistibly to London. The winter term at St Bartholomew's was about to begin and, although he now had no formal association with the Hospital, he still felt it to be his spiritual home. His father decided to allow him £10 per month until he became self-supporting, on the understanding that he would return home at the end of six months, if by then he had no definite prospects. When James later said that he 'drifted rather than sailed or steered back to London' he was probably recalling his lack of any clear idea as to how he would keep himself.

He took rooms in Millman Street and began to earn a small income by teaching groups of medical students who were preparing for their examinations. These young men were willing to pay for short cuts to knowledge and hints on easy ways to remember dull facts. This 'grinding' was a form of teaching that Paget did not enjoy, or do well, but he desperately needed the money. One student, 'a quiet, gentlemanly fellow', boarded with him, paying £10 per month. By such means Paget could manage to be largely independent of his father.

James becomes engaged

No sooner were these arrangements complete than he took a step that amazed the family. He announced his engagement to Miss Lydia North, the daughter of the clergyman who had been so hospitable to him during his student days. James later recalled:

> It would have been difficult to do anything not immoral which could have seemed to any reasonable person more imprudent; and it is not to be pretended that wisdom, discretion, fore-thought, or any method of sound judgment, had anything to do with it; I had been for nearly two years falling in love and now suddenly confessed it and was believed trustworthy. The indis-cretion was the happiest event of my life: the beginning of an engagement which for nearly eight years gave me help and hope enough to make even the heaviest work seem light, and then ended in a marriage blest with constancy of perfect mutual love not once disturbed. No human wisdom could have devised a step so wise as was this rash engagement.[1]

Mr North evidently approved of James as a prospective son-in-law, but Samuel Paget was outspoken in his opposition to the en-gagement. He wrote to Henry North:

> I find by a letter from my son James that he has made an offer to your amiable daughter & that you are also made acquainted with his having done so. I think it therefore only my duty to write you on the subject, not with the intention, I assure you to interfere with the sentiments of the parties, but to urge most strongly the inexpediency, & indeed the impropriety of our allowing our two young people to contract an engagement which cannot be fulfilled perhaps for half a dozen years—with my family and the demand for the completion of their education I can allow James nothing. He has now another year of probation & after that I shall be at a loss to know where he can set down to prosecute his profession, every town being full of medical prac-titioners. I have written most unreservedly as I know you like that best, and, I repeat, I do hope & trust for all our sakes, you will urge the inexpediency of this matter going on . . .[2]

James's brothers and sisters were equally hostile to the engage-ment. They thought him both irresponsible and disloyal to the family. They even refused to welcome Lydia as a future sister-in-law. But the young couple were not discouraged and the engage-ment continued. The episode could have resulted in a permanent rift between James and the rest of his family, but it did not do so. The letters that were exchanged between London, Yarmouth, and

Cambridge, as freely as ever, contained views on every subject of mutual interest other than the engagement. James refused to discuss this intensely personal matter, preferring to wait for his opponents' attitude to change with the passage of time. Gradually the family came to accept that he did not intend to rush headlong into marriage, but was prepared to wait until he was able to support a wife. Even so, it was some years before they could bring themselves to refer to James's fiancee as 'Lydia' rather than 'Miss North'. The ability to withstand opposition patiently and without bitterness was one of James Paget's characteristics, and one that would soon be tested again.

Controversy over Paget's first appointment at St Bartholomew's

In November Mr Bayntin, 'the very neat and careful dissector', announced that he would resign from the post of Curator of the Hospital museum in the following spring. Through the influence of Mr Stanley the position was offered to Paget. The Curator's salary was only £100 per year but, added to his income from teaching, it would free him from any reliance on his father. At St Bartholomew's the post of Curator was considered a minor one, although at several other London hospitals similar appointments carried higher status and were held by eminent men. Before accepting, Paget asked that the additional title of Assistant Demonstrator of Anatomy be added to that of Curator. This would not increase his salary, but would probably lead, in due course, to his becoming Demonstrator of Anatomy. In the past, Demonstrators of Anatomy had usually become Assistant Surgeons. Stanley was eager to have Paget as Curator of the museum, but he balked at giving him the second title because of the controversy it would provoke. His colleagues would see it as an attempt to break the tradition that surgical appointments were given only to former apprentices of Hospital surgeons. Stanley suggested, instead, the title of Demonstrator of Morbid Anatomy. This carried less status and was not a direct path to a surgical appointment. But even here Paget met with opposition, this time from Thomas Wormald, the popular Senior Demonstrator. Between Paget and Wormald, who was 'a shrewd, hard-headed Yorkshireman', there was a natural antipathy. As a student, Paget was disgusted by Wormald's use of obscene jokes to enliven his anatomy demonstrations and had made no secret of his feelings. Now Wormald retaliated by opposing the extension of any favours to Paget. So Paget had to be content with the simple title of Curator. At least he would have a salary and an official position at the Hospital. The family at Yarmouth drank a toast in his honour and sent him their congratulations.

The negotiations over the appointment had dragged on for a

month. A more pleasant episode that occurred during this period helped to revive Paget's spirits. Dr Marshall Hall, the renowned physiologist, knew of his translations of recent papers by the German scientist Johannes Muller; he invited Paget to call on him so that they could discuss Muller's views on spinal reflexes. The meeting was cordial and of benefit to both men. In the course of conversation Marshall Hall mentioned that he hoped to establish a new medical school and that, if he succeeded, he would invite his guest to join the staff. Paget's ambitions were still centred on St Bartholomew's Hospital, but he appreciated the compliment.

Time spent with his family is followed by a study tour to Paris

After the meeting with Marshall Hall Paget changed his plans for the four months he had to fill in before his duties as Curator began. He decided to terminate the irksome 'grinding' classes, return home for Christmas, and then depart for the Continent. In Paris he could live very cheaply, while attending lectures and ward rounds conducted by some internationally famous men. Large numbers of students from Europe and North America flocked to Paris to hear these men, but Paget would probably not have such an opportunity again for a number of years.

The celebration of Christmas in the house on the Quay was as joyful as the family could make it. To add to their anxieties, in October Mrs Paget had suffered a serious illness, which Charles Costerton ascribed to some mushrooms she had eaten. Within a few days she was out of danger, but her convalescence was protracted and by Christmas she still had not recovered her former robust health.

James's correspondence with Lydia during this period of separation was his defence against loneliness. From Yarmouth he wrote an account of a particularly severe storm that left dozens of ships wrecked on the Norfolk coast:

> . . . You can conceive nothing more terrible than the gale which has now been blowing since Saturday morning from the E. and N.E. Directly after church yesterday, hearing that some vessels were on shore, I went down to the beach—the wind was blowing a perfect hurricane, the sea rushing in the most appalling power and velocity, and covered as it were with one surface of boiling foam. Two vessels, out of many that were in the Roads, were already on the beach; and as I stood there, another was blown on—the others were all pitching most frightfully. In another hour, two more came on: one of them had just time to set her sails, and made an attempt to get into the Harbour. It was intensely exciting—she had been driven almost into the breakers, but as

they got up her topsails and put her helm down she bounded off with the speed as it were of lightening, and with her decks almost under water she flew over the billows. We could follow her as she went, and saw her apparently enter the harbour—everything seemed safe—but at last she checked in her course, and presently her foremast fell overboard: she had missed the river, and gone on to the beach in the South Haven: she is by this time a perfect wreck.

Most providentially it was high tide, and but few of the vessels were laden, so that they are washed very high up on the beach, and all their crews were saved with but little difficulty. At night between 10 and 11 I went down again: the wind was not in the slightest degree abated, and there was then a heavy fall of snow. Three more vessels were on shore—one had struck the jetty, driving-in several of the piles, and was now lying beaten against it. I never saw so awful a scene in my life—the end of the jetty was almost constantly under water from the seas repeatedly washing over it, and the moon was completely obscured by the clouds of snow that were falling. You could hear nothing but the tremendous roaring of the wind among the ropes and tattered sails of the vessels as they lay on the beach. I walked down again this morning before breakfast—the destruction was increased and still increasing. I left no fewer than fifteen fine vessels on shore within three miles of the jetty: and the sea is still as high as ever. The crews are all, however, by God's mercy saved, and many of the vessels will probably not sustain much damage— but, if the gale continue, their number will be even further fearfully increased.[3]

It was late in January when he set off for Paris. The channel crossing was uneventful apart from his being asked to help a woman in labour. Paget successfully 'ushered into the world a young sea-nymph' and when the ship arrived at Boulogne mother and child were both in excellent condition. His first letter from Paris was dated Jan. 29th, 1837—

After an hour's ineffectual attempts at lighting a fire on two logs of damp wood, I may surely take refuge in writing to you. Try to imagine me, sitting in a low chair, at a high table, in a room about 12 feet square, at once my chamber and drawing room, without a carpet, or anything presenting the smallest appearance of comfort—and to add to my chagrin the only *garçon* on the establishment who is not enjoying the gaieties of the Sunday has just shown me that it was simply my ignorance of wood-fires that prevented my lighting it. Well, well! It is not after all essential to one's happiness to be secure from these small annoyances, and I thank God I have too many blessings to allow them to occupy more than a small share of my attention.[4]

But he did not succumb to the enchantment of Paris. Perhaps his personal circumstances, rather than the city, were to blame. He was miserably short of money, worried about his future, and, worst of all, he was lonely. He seemed to feel aggressively Protestant, even Puritanical, when he found himself in the midst of pre-Lenten merrymaking.

> The Sunday before Lent is here called *Dimanche Gras,* being celebrated by a grand procession round the most public parts of Paris to exhibit a Fat Ox. . . . The *Boeuf Gras* was not larger than a moderately good Hereford Ox; and the procession was most absurd. Nothing could be more utterly French than the Carnival itself. The whole of the Boulevards, for about six miles in extent, were crowded with people in carriages and on foot, to see a few fools in costumes and masques—it was the most extraordinary case of one fool making many I ever saw, and does as little credit to their decency as to their taste, seeing that the persons whom the better class, and in fact all Paris, went to see and mix with, were of course not even of doubtful morality. The costumes were (at least in Public) very poor; and indeed nothing but gross buffoonery seemed to be aimed at. At night, the streets were full of people going to about 80 different masked balls; and next morning (that of Ash Wednesday) there were hundreds of men and women reeling intoxicated about the streets, attempting to go home from the night's orgies. It was a perfect scene of public dissipation and bestiality. I remained at home nearly the whole day, to cleanse myself of the pollution.[5]

Fortunately the carnival was soon over and the sober atmosphere of Lent made it easier for him to pursue his medical studies. He attended lectures by the leading men in the profession, including his hero, the anatomist Cloquet. Of the teaching in the hospitals, he found much to praise, but also much that merited criticism:

> The state of medical science in France is on the whole, I should say, very nearly equal to that which it has attained in England. In many points, especially in surgical practice, they are far inferior; in others, as the science of medicine, they are far superior—though I question whether this be not the merely temporary effect of the coincidence of three or four highly talented men, who give their attention to it exclusively. In their knowledge of the works of others, or in what we call medical learning, they are

far inferior to all other nations; so that perhaps their numerous piracies are excusable on the ground of ignorance. For the study of medicine, generally and in all its branches, their plan is on the whole inferior to the English: the very excess of means which they possess in some parts makes them superficial in all; while in others, and especially in Hospital practice, they have scarcely any opportunity of studying at all; and hence I do not doubt the fact of their inferiority as practitioners. On the other hand, the advantages they offer to any one who wishes to study any one class of disease in particular are immense; and they deserve great blame for not having made far better use of them.[6]

But his visit was not without its happy moments. He allowed himself some minor indulgences which, in London, he would have thought too frivolous; he attended a performance by a popular actress, witnessed a debate in the Chamber of Deputies, and heard the controversial preacher Père Lacordaire. He read Pascal's *Pensées* for the first time, and was profoundly moved. But by far the most enjoyable experience was a two-day walking excursion in the forest of Fontainebleau, with a party of four English friends. He wrote to Lydia: 'I never wished more to have you with me, and I think, if we are spared to tourize together, our first trip shall be to Fontainebleau—even though it be necessary to go to it through Paris.'

Medical journalism supplements his income as Curator
In April, 1837, Paget returned to London and his old lodgings in Millman Street. Shortly afterwards he took up his post as Curator.

The work of the place was hard, and some of it rather menial. In most of the years, I had to be at the Museum from 9 to 4 on every day but Saturday; and to put-up all new specimens, and keep in order all the old ones, and to take care that Stanley had, in their due places, all the illustrations that he needed for his lectures— diagrams, preparations, and the rest. And sketches had to be made for him; hideous, rectilinear things, enough to spoil one's eyes. Besides, I had to manage all things connected with the supply of subjects for dissection, and to put-up all notices of lectures, and see to the printing of the Students' Guide-book, and many other pieces of job-work.[7]

Another of his duties as Curator was the preparation of a new catalogue of the Hospital museum. The first catalogue, which had been compiled some years earlier by Edward Stanley, had been rendered obsolete by the addition of new specimens and by changes to the system of classification. This task was to occupy part of nearly every working day of Paget's life for the next nine years.

He still needed additional sources of income. He decided against taking another resident pupil, the indolence of the first having been a constant source of irritation, but he did resume his classes for examination candidates. Another type of work that he undertook proved to be much more interesting; he became a medical journalist.

> I used to earn from this work from £50 to £70 a year; and I have always been glad to have known the work of a journalist, and to remember how much less it is either influential or contemptible than those are apt to think who know nothing of it. It is good to know the kind of men that are reviewers; good to be able to estimate fairly, in after-life, the weight of their praise or blame; and to be quite sure that this weight is never great. And there is a use in being required, sometimes, to write off-hand about something half-known: it helps to give an ability which, like that for being crammed, is very valuable, provided only it be rarely exercised and kept rigidly under restraint. There is use, too, in learning to report from memory, as, for about two years, I reported the debates at the Medico-Chirurgical Society; not by taking notes, but by listening attentively and writing-down at home the chief things said. I can clearly trace some of my facility in the work of after-life to the having been on the staff of a journal.[8]

Paget was associated with two journals—the *Medical Gazette* and the *Medical Quarterly Review*. From 1837 to 1842 he was sub-editor of the *Gazette* which, unlike its crusading contemporary, the *Lancet,* was 'a completely respectable and rather dull journal'. He wrote many of its leading articles and also contributed translations of papers that had appeared in the French and German scientific press. Many years later, Paget described his leading articles for the *Gazette* as 'generally discreet, not lively or clever, very rarely political, chiefly on questions of medical education, on scientific progress, discoveries, and the like.'

The work for the *Quarterly Review* was more demanding. The *Review*'s editor was Dr John Forbes (later Sir John Forbes) who aimed to make the journal a forum for the leading men in medical science. In 1821 Forbes had produced the first English translation of the writings of Laennec, in which the invention of the stethoscope and its use in the examination of the chest are described. Forbes thereby associated himself with the new medical philosophy, in which the first task of the physician became that of making an accurate diagnosis. This was based partly on the patient's history and partly on the findings at a careful physical examination. He showed how, with the aid of the stethoscope, it was possible to detect subtle abnormal signs, signs that were clues to the nature of diseases of the heart and lungs. Many of Forbes's contemporaries were sceptical; some regarded the stethoscope as a useless toy. Forbes countered by publishing in the *Review* reports of the progress being made by men who shared his opinions.

Paget's association with the *Review*, begun in 1837, continued for many years. At first he was conscious of an onerous responsibility; for each *Review* article he wrote, he read every significant article on the subject, not only in English, but in French, German, and Italian. The gain to himself in breadth of knowledge was a reward, but there were also other benefits from his contacts with medical journalists. He became well known, not only to Forbes, but also to James Clark, Forbes's life-long friend. Clark had been physician to the Duchess of Kent, the mother of Princess Victoria. The young Princess became Queen in July, 1837. She appointed Clark her physician-in-ordinary, and three months later honoured him with a baronetcy. Although Paget never consciously sought the favour of men in high places, he freely acknowledged in later life that his career had benefitted from his association with influential men like Forbes and Clark.

Paget's third commitment as a journalist was to an organisation known as the Society for the Diffusion of Useful Knowledge. This body had been formed in 1826 by Henry Brougham, who, in 1830, became Lord Brougham, Lord Chancellor of England. Brougham had outstanding talents as a jurist and an orator, but his somewhat eccentric personality marred his political career. Among his many interests were two that were always dear to his heart—the anti-slavery campaign, and the movement for the provision of better education for the poor. In forming the Society for the Diffusion of Useful knowledge he had the support of forty-seven public-spirited gentlemen, fifteen of whom were Fellows of the Royal Society. Brougham's group undertook the publication of inexpensive books, journals, and maps, on subjects of general interest and practical importance, 'for the imparting of useful knowledge to all classes of the community, particularly such as are unable to avail themselves of experienced teachers, or may prefer learning by themselves.' One of their most successful publications was the *Penny Magazine*, which was later converted to the *Penny Cyclopaedia*. In 1842 the Society began a biographical dictionary. This was planned on a very ambitious scale and proved too costly for the Society's limited resources. Its publication had to cease when only the first seven volumes, covering the letter A, had been produced. Of his work for the *Penny Cyclopaedia* and the *Biographical Dictionary* Paget wrote:

The writers for both these works (and they included many of the best of the time) had the advantage of working under a remarkably good editor, George Long. His own proper range was in classics, and ancient law: but he had in a high degree that singular power of widely-ranging good editors which enables them to detect errors or doubtful points in essays on subjects of which they know, of their own study, little or nothing. Nothing written lightly or carelessly ever seemed to escape him. It was for me an excellent exercise in accuracy—and in writing biographies—though the Dictionary came to an end at the close of letter A, in its 7th volume, and was said to have exhausted both the patience and the funds of the Society. The work was in an entirely new field, and had to be done in what was to me a nearly new manner—with the reading of old books, and the searching everywhere in old journals, and the Transactions of old Societies, and tracking my way for references anywhere, so as to have at least a nearly complete list of every considerable writer's works. I had, before this, known very little of the history of medicine: I ended with knowing not much more, but with a clear impression of the immense difficulty of writing an accurate and nearly complete history of any time or science; and with a thorough disregard for all histories written lightly or prettily. Besides, I learnt more than ever the value or necessity of always referring, if possible, to the very book, volume, and page quoted from, or from which any statement is made, and the similar necessity of verifying every reference made from another. Nothing could better teach the difficulty, necessity, and rarity of accuracy in writing than did this work in biography.[9]

Such a cool appraisal of the benefits derived from his work as a journalist was possible for the elderly gentleman writing his memoirs, but at the time he had been more conscious of the meagre, but vital, financial rewards, as this letter to George Paget, written in May, 1838, shows:

My present prospects and conditions in money matters are not bad. The next number (monthly) of the 'Penny Cyclopaedia' will contain about £25 worth of mine . . . This is an unusual haul—still, I think I may calculate on £70 a year from it while it lasts. I can work the Gazette to about £80 a year more; so that I may, I hope, reckon on £200 a year, which will swim me.[10]

It sometimes troubled Paget that he had to devote so much of his time to writing. When he left the Hospital museum each day, instead of being able to visit the wards he had to spend many hours in the library of the Royal College of Surgeons, or at the British Museum, gathering material for his articles. As a student he had been denied practical surgical experience; now his writing activities were perpetuating the problem. There was a danger that he could be permanently excluded from the surgical career that was his real objective.

Still working long hours and living frugally
He now earned enough to be self-supporting, but he was also anxious to help the family at Yarmouth. He sent them his small savings and at times borrowed money to tide his father over a crisis. He lived frugally and worked long hours every day; an evening's relaxation had to be paid for by working until 3 a.m. the next night. To save money he regularly went without dinner on Fridays, and chewed dates and raisins to appease his hunger. It was not surprising that he became ill from time to time. In August, 1837, he suffered from pneumonia; this was the first of many attacks of this disease he had in succeeding years.

In January, 1838, Paget moved to new lodgings at 3, Serle Street, Lincoln's Inn Fields. He hoped to attract fee-paying patients from among the legal fraternity of Lincoln's Inn, one of the four Inns of Court. His rooms were above Ravenscroft's shop, where barristers' wigs and gowns were sold. He had

> a front-room, decently furnished, and a back-room furnished with only a turn-up bedstead and a washing-stand. One room was sufficient for the practice, which was, on an average, £13 or £14 a year; and I never had two patients at a time; and visitors were so rare that a furnished waiting-room was quite unnecessary.[11]

In the same month an assistant-surgeon appointment was to be made at the Hospital, and Paget entered the contest, although he knew he had no chance of succeeding. Canvassing by candidates, as for a political election, was the accepted practice. For ten days he curtailed his writing activities in order to visit the Hospital Governors and present his credentials. Shortly before the closing date he withdrew from the contest. The appointment went to Thomas Wormald. In a letter to George, James explained that the time and effort had been well spent, since he had established his right to be considered as a candidate, even though he was not a former Hospital apprentice. He felt optimistic that in due course he would succeed.

Death and disappointment
Events later in the year tested his courage. In March his good friend Johnstone contracted 'typhus'—the distinction between typhus and typhoid was not then recognized. Both conditions at times became epidemic among the poor, because of their crowded, unsani-

tary living conditions. The organism responsible for typhoid is a bacterium that spreads from human to human when food or water becomes contaminated with infected excreta. The typhus organism, which is even smaller than a bacterium, is spread by body lice. An epidemic of one of these diseases had broken out in London six months previously, and over 150 cases were treated at St Bartholomew's Hospital. There had been several deaths among Hospital staff. Johnstone was one in whom the disease ran a fulminating course; he died in the second week of his illness. James wrote to George:

> Poor Johnstone died last night: he had never rallied from the commencement of the attack, but, as long as his senses remained, despairing of recovery, he went on from bad to worse with scarcely a hope. He had been most carefully attended by Drs Hue and Budd, but medicine had no influence whatever on the disease, which seemed to *poison* him. I cannot tell you how I feel his loss—he was the only friend I had in the Hospital, and he was a most sincere and estimable one. I had never received anything but the truest pleasure and profit from his society, and I shall look in vain for someone to fill up the perfect loneliness in which I now find myself left here. The loss to his family will be fearful— from what his sister told me he seems to have been their only stay.[12]

Two months later Paget suffered another blow. His salary as Curator was reduced from £100 to £40. The reasons given were that the Curator should devote the whole of his time to the work, and should also give an undertaking to remain in the position for a number of years. Paget would not accept either of these conditions, so his salary was reduced. He believed that he owed this misfortune to the ill-will of one member of the staff, whom he did not name, but who was probably Wormald. The lower salary was, however, coupled with shorter working hours: in future he would attend the Museum only from 12 to 4 each day. At first the financial loss seemed almost more than he could bear, but even more hurtful was the malevolence of the person responsible. Paget entertained the idea of leaving St Bartholomew's and joining the Aldersgate Street school. On further reflection he decided to make the best of his truncated appointment. The extra time at his disposal could be put to good use, and there was a reasonable chance that he could make up the lost income by extra writing.

He was familiar with the work of Bichat, the French anatomist who died in 1802. Bichat had introduced the concept of 'general anatomy', in which the descriptions are based on systems, such as the nervous and vascular systems, rather than regions, such as the abdomen or the lower limb. General anatomy provided a useful basis for the study of physiology, and was regarded as a significant advance. Paget had already begun work on his own textbook of general anatomy when his appointment as Curator was curtailed. He resolved that thereafter he would devote several extra hours each day to his book. Successful publication of such a work would add to his reputation and would also provide some income.

Serious illness
On 18 December, 1838, Paget carried out a post-mortem examination in a slum dwelling in Lambeth. The subject was a woman who had been living in wretched poverty, and was shortly to have gone to a workhouse. She had been found dead in her bed on the floor. Nine cases of 'typhus' (in this instance probably true typhus) had recently occurred in the same dwelling, although the woman's death was due to another cause. Nevertheless Paget evidently contracted typhus while working in the vermin-infested house. He went home to Yarmouth to spend Christmas with his family, and noticed the first symptoms on 29 December, the day on which he began the journey back to London. He became ill during the fifteen-hour coach journey and by the time he reached his lodgings his condition was serious. His kindly landlady took care of him and summoned the aid of his family. George and Charles hastened to London and together, with the landlady's assistance, they nursed him through the crisis. Their anxiety must have been heightened by their awareness of the fate of James's friend Johnstone. On 5 January George wrote home to Alfred:

James's illness has run a most dangerous course, but thanks be to God it now appears to have taken a favourable turn. I believe I am not too sanguine in considering that it has passed its worst crisis. Every thing that care can effect shall be done to prevent a relapse. Poor fellow—at 12 last night we thought he was dying, and indeed no living man could be nearer to it. The favourable change showed itself at 5 A.M. You shall hear regularly of him in future. Offer your prayers and thanks to God for this appearance of recovery.[13]

Charles's letter of 23 January tells of the patient's convalescence:

Yesterday, he got up, with some assistance; and on my arm he came and *breakfasted with me* in his sitting-room, blanketted and pillowed in an easy chair, sat a little while afterwards and then to bed, and up again to dinner with me, and after a bit of Yarmouth chicken drank all your good healths in a glass of (a little diluted) port—and to bed again. If it pleases God to continue this great mercy to him and us, I think in a week from this time you may be looking out to see us. Tomorrow we shall drink your healths at a much earlier hour, James' appetite for dinner being quite prepared and ready by one. He is sporting a new wig—I tell him 'tis a judgment for wearing his own hair so badly—wig rather curly. I do not wonder at his exertion to get-on up here. For medical men, what a difference! I never saw such agreeable and talented men as all who visit him—Dr. Latham (who asked after you), Dr. Burrows, &c. &c. The first-named, when I thanked him for his kindness to James, his reply was most satisfactory—'Oh, don't talk about it: he is a most valuable man, and will continue to be, to his fellow-creatures.'[14]

The boredom of Paget's convalescence must have been relieved by an incident that was the talk of London's medical and social circles. It was generally known that the young Queen had only with difficulty freed herself from the domination of her mother, the Duchess of Kent. The Duchess was aided and supported by her maid-of-honour, Lady Flora Hastings. Consequently relations between the Queen and Lady Flora were strained.

In January, 1839, Lady Flora, who was thirty-three years old, consulted Sir James Clark because she was suffering from vague ill-health, associated with abdominal swelling and discomfort. She declined to undergo a physical examination, so Sir James could do nothing more than prescribe symptomatic treatment. As her abdominal swelling increased the Court began to buzz with rumours that the unmarried Lady Flora was pregnant. The Queen, incensed at her adversary's apparent flaunting of her condition, instructed her Prime Minister, Lord Melbourne, to investigate the matter. Melbourne asked Clark if it was true that Lady Flora was pregnant, but the physician could only reply that he did not know. Melbourne would have preferred to let the matter rest, but the Queen insisted that it be resolved as soon as possible. Reluctantly, Melbourne persuaded Clark to convey to Lady Flora the message that it was virtually a royal command that she submit to a medical examination. She agreed to be examined by Sir James and her own family physician, Sir Charles Clarke. The two doctors subsequently issued a statement, dated 17 February, 1839:

We have examined, with great care, the state of Lady Flora Hastings, with a view to determine the existence or non-existence of pregnancy, and it is our opinion, although there is an enlargement of the stomach, that there are no grounds for suspicion that pregnancy does exist or ever did exist.[15]

Within a few weeks it was obvious that Lady Flora was seriously ill. The abdominal swelling increased, jaundice developed, and she became emaciated. She died in July, 1839. A post-mortem examination revealed that death was due to liver disease; it also confirmed that she had never been pregnant.

Lady Flora's indignant relatives wrote to *The Times,* complaining of the ill-treatment their kinswoman had received at Court. Of course the Queen was not named, but the implication that she was at fault was obvious. The incident caused a sharp, though temporary, decline in the popularity of both the Queen and her Prime Minister. Sir James Clark's professional reputation also suffered. Court gossip held that he had misdiagnosed Lady Flora's condition as pregnancy at the first consultation, and that he, therefore, was responsible for the whole unpleasant misunderstanding. Sir James had acted entirely within the precepts of his generation of medical men; nevertheless his practice declined sharply, and remained in this state for several years.

The incident stimulated public debate on the relationship between doctor and patient. Clearly it was unreasonable for any patient to expect her physician to treat her without allowing him to make a physical examination. Should Sir James Clark have refused to prescribe under these circumstances? And what of the confidentiality that should exist between doctor and patient? Perhaps not even the sovereign should have been allowed to breach this for reasons that were not of national importance. Paget would have been interested in the broader implications of the controversy. Doctors were being asked to accept greater responsibility for their patients' welfare; to do this they needed to be trusted and respected. Their patients could not expect them to pander to their whims as their hairdressers and dressmakers did.

Meanwhile, George Paget's career was progressing satisfactorily. In 1838 he was awarded the MD, Cambridge; a year later he became a Fellow of the Royal College of Physicians and was elected Physician to Addenbrooke's Hospital, Cambridge. Just as James was to remain all his life a 'Bart's man', so was George dedicated to the service of Addenbrooke's Hospital and Cambridge University. George was not physically strong. He suffered from recurrent attacks of rheumatic fever that interrupted his work but, even so, he continued to advance professionally and in the esteem of his friends.

Demonstratorship leads to lecturing

The Demonstratorship in Morbid Anatomy, which James Paget had been denied in 1836, was offered to him in the summer of 1839; he accepted it gladly. Despite its title, it was not then regarded as a teaching appointment, the holder's duties being limited to the performance of post-mortem examinations on Hospital patients. But within a few months a group of students made a formal request for lectures on morbid anatomy, to be given by Mr Paget. (Among the signatories to the request were George Murray Humphry and Anthony Brownless. Humphry later became Professor of Anatomy at Cambridge and helped to make this a medical school of world renown. Brownless migrated to Australia in 1852; he was appointed chairman of a committee that established the medical faculty of Melbourne University.)

The students' request met with opposition. Some of the senior staff members saw it as yet another attempt by Paget, the outsider, to encroach on the privileges reserved for Hospital apprentices. But they had no other teacher of morbid anatomy whose knowledge of the subject could rival Paget's. Furthermore, the popularity of St Bartholomew's medical school had been steadily declining because of its lack of gifted teachers. The Governors knew that unless they remedied this deficiency the school would not survive. The request was granted.

At first Paget was restricted to using the post-mortem room, where the students had to stand, but in the following year he was granted the use of the anatomy lecture theatre. The lectures were a great success:

These were the first lectures that I ever gave; and they were well attended, though they were neither compulsory nor paid-for. They gave me the best possible opportunity for practice in lecturing; for I adopted the plan, then not usual, of lecturing on the specimens obtained in *post-mortem* examinations of the day or few days before, neglecting all attempts at systematic teaching, and describing or explaining little more than could be shown to the naked eye or be touched. I have no doubt that this is the best plan of teaching pathological anatomy to students; certainly it was the best for me; for there was not time enough for either learning the lectures or so writing them that they might be in part or wholly read. I was compelled to speak extemporaneously, unless, it might be, in some chief sentences which could be learned by heart. I never had difficulty in thus speaking; but the practice, and the repute which some success in it gave me, were of immense value; the more, probably, because the lectures were popular with the students and of some use, perhaps, in checking the decline of the school and in making my superiors think that I deserved something more lucrative—though, indeed, I still feel well enough repaid by the possession of a handsome silver tea-service, and a largely-signed address, and by the memory of the very good dinner at which these were presented.[16]

Although Paget here commends the extemporaneous style of delivery, his reputation as a speaker later in his career reflected his skill in using the opposite approach. His formal addresses and lectures were prepared so carefully, and he took such pains to be familiar with his material, that he could deliver even a long oration almost without the aid of notes.

As well as establishing him as a lecturer, the Demonstratorship brought other rewards. The performance of a large number of post-mortem examinations gave him opportunities for making the kind of original observations that had led to his *Trichina* discovery. He noticed that many of the adult patients who died in the Hospital had dull white patches in the pericardium, the normally smooth and glistening membrane that covers the surface of the heart. These patches were sometimes found in the absence of any other indication that the patient had suffered from heart disease. James first mentioned his discovery in a letter to Lydia North written in July, 1839. In November he presented his findings at a meeting of the Medico-Chirurgical Society, and thus made his second contribution to medical literature. His paper was entitled *On White Spots on the Surface of the Heart, and on the Frequency of Pericarditis.* Later generations of medical students have had to learn the numerous causes of pericarditis, and that many of these are not primarily diseases of the heart.

A Spartan existence relieved by Lydia and his family
Work continued to occupy almost all of his time. Although fond of congenial company and good conversation, he had of necessity reduced his circle of friends to the very few for whom he had a deep regard. His letters to Lydia and to his family provided him with a means of self-expression and communication with the outside world, without which he could not have borne his Spartan existence. In a letter to Lydia, dated 19 August, 1840, he wrote:

> I do think I have succeeded to perfection in offending most of my useless acquaintance. I can scarcely remember my last invitation to an Evening-party; and, so far as I can judge, I have less prospect than ever of their being repeated—It is really a great deliverance from anxiety and trouble; and if it leaves me more disposed and more at leisure for your society, you dearest at least can have no reason to complain. I fear you will think that in spite of your kind remonstrances I am still growing more unsocial.[17]

From time to time members of his family would stay with him for a few days when they had to come to London. Frank, especially, was good company. Although an energetic worker, Frank could always put aside his cares briefly if an opportunity arose to enjoy some new experience. Then he would write graphic letters to the family describing all that he had seen. Frank made one such visit to London in June, 1841. James was unable to leave his work, so Frank went sight-seeing by himself. He enjoyed the spectacle of the crowds at the races on Derby Day. Next day he went on a trip to Windsor, and was involved in a train accident. He wrote of all this to Alfred:

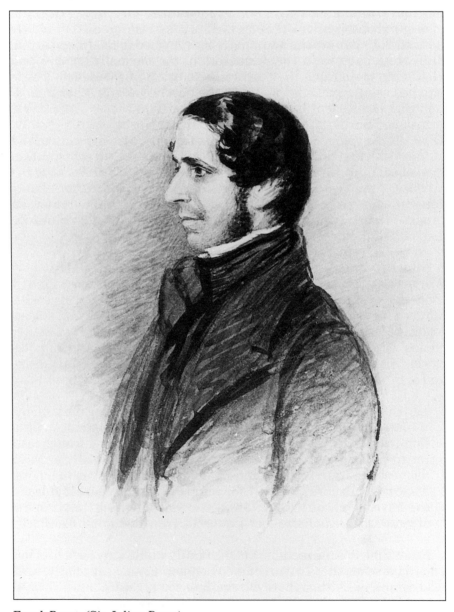

Frank Paget. (Sir Julian Paget).

I, next day, although expecting James to go with me, went down to Windsor to see the Castle, with a letter of introduction from John Crome to Stark, the Artist, and French, a chorister. I went by the Great Western Railway. Oh, what beautiful travelling in the First Class carriages, and only 4/6. James was prevented going on account of three bodies he had to cut up. Well, we got to Slough in 35 minutes, and then I rode on the box of an omnibus to Windsor. Oh superb, the finest day possible, things smelling deliciously; passed Eton, a perfect heaven the drive from Eton to Windsor Castle. After taking a chop with Stark, and looking at his pictures, which were very good, all in the old Crome style, we started for the Castle. Well, my dear Alfred, the *pictures,* tapestry, drawing rooms, St. George's Hall, the *Waterloo* Gallery, the suits of gold armour, the Banners of all the Knights, and so on! Now comes my journey back to Town. Thanks be to God for preserving me to relate all this. Only conceive, an accident on the Railway about 15 miles from London. The engine broke down, caught fire, and burst its pipes, half drowning us all, as I went up in a second class carriage, therefore open. Our first announcement was the pipes of water, playing on our backs drenching all to the skin. Then after 5 minutes we stopped, women fainting, men calling out etc., begging to guards to unlock the doors. After a long time they let us out; I went to look at the engine; there were the stokers and the engineers, looking like devils, half naked, taking up the gravel and endeavouring to put the fire out. Well, the fear was the train coming on the same line behind us. The guard ran back and hoisted up the signals of an accident, a red, green and white light. This stopped them, and in about an hour they came up and pushed us before them at about 5 miles an hour. I was frightened so much that I thought of walking up to Town with 3 or 4 more passengers. We were going, when the pipe burst, 50 miles an hour, as we were ten minutes behind time. I forgot to say that, going from the place where the Star stopped, Chevallier and myself got spilt in a cab, nobody of course hurt: the Police came up and soon put us to rights.[18]

Two days later he inspected the Tower of London, then joined the crowds waiting to see the Members leaving the House of Lords.

They said the Duke of Wellington would soon come. I had not been there ten minutes before out he came and rode past me with his brother. . . . What do you think of this for a sight! I was looked at by the Duke, whom I took off my hat to; he touched his in return. He is getting very old, and every two minutes kept opening his mouth, not speaking. But oh, what thoughts came into my mind as I walked beside him! Oh, what a soldier! How he sat his horse while he talked with his brother![19]

In a few days Frank had done more sight-seeing than James had in seven years.

Vigorous canvassing wins a position at the Finsbury Dispensary

In April, 1841, Paget learned of a vacancy on the staff of the Finsbury Dispensary; since he greatly needed clinical practice, he decided to apply. The Dispensary treated out-patients drawn from the local population of labourers and crafstmen and their families. His attendance would be required for three mornings a week, an arrangement that was quite compatible with his duties as Curator at the Hospital. But even this relatively humble appointment was not to be won without a struggle. Vigorous canvassing was essential and Paget was a late entrant. Sir James Clark came to his aid and Paget was elected with a comfortable majority.

In 1841 it seemed that his period of hardship was about to end. Thomas Wormald announced his intention of resigning from the Hospital, and Stanley nominated Paget to succeed Wormald as Demonstrator of Anatomy. The additional salary of £100 would have been enough to solve all Paget's immediate problems and would even have made it possible for him to marry. Furthermore, an appointment as Assistant-Surgeon to the Hospital would almost certainly have followed. Paget's joy was short-lived. There were vehement protests from nineteen apprentices, all of whom were seeking Hospital appointments. They were supported by a section of the students, who preferred Wormald's practical and racy style as a lecturer to that of the quiet and scholarly Paget. So Wormald was pursuaded to withdraw his resignation and the offer to Paget was cancelled.

The loss of the Demonstratorship was a bitter disappointment; for years Paget kept as a memento his copy of the terms under which it had been offered. But despite this defeat, he could sense that the apprenticeship system was coming to an end, and that his own reputation at the Hospital was steadily growing. Good news from home at this time also helped to cheer him. His father was honoured at a festival held by the shipping clubs of Yarmouth. Samuel Paget had been a member for forty-five years, and served as treasurer of his club for twenty-five years. In 1841 the clubs were about to be reorganized, and before losing their original identities they decided to reward one of their longest serving and most loyal supporters. Samuel Paget was guest of honour at a dinner for 130 clubmen. After the speeches he was presented with a magnificent silver soup tureen. James could not be there, but he received a detailed account of the occasion in letters from the family. To his mother he wrote in reply:

I have been looking anxiously for some account (in the newspapers) of the Paget *fête,* which I cannot but regard as the highest honour which my father, in his position, is capable of having attained. If he had set himself, when young, the highest earthly object which a Merchant in Yarmouth could hope to attain, it might well have been this which he reached on Thursday. But enough of this—I do not doubt he had compliments enough paid him to last him for many a long year. May God grant him many an one; and make us feel the responsibility that lies on us to maintain his good name . . .[20]

At other times letters from home contained reports of the sad decline in his mother's health. The acute illness that had been ascribed to poisonous mushrooms had left her permanently weakened and with a progressive disability. Her vision was slowly deteriorating, her speech becoming slurred. The once busy hands were losing their strength and co-ordination. Her mind was as alert and bright as ever, and she still wrote frequently to the sons who were away from home, but the change in her handwriting told them quite clearly of her increasing invalidism. The two daughters, Patty and Kate, gradually took over the tasks of household management as they became too much for their mother's declining powers.

The Royal College of Surgeons and the Hunterian Museum
In 1842 Paget was asked by the Council of the Royal College of Surgeons to compile a descriptive catalogue of the specimens in the Hunterian Museum. This was not just a mundane task, but one of considerable importance, since the College's function as a teaching body had helped to shape its history. When Henry VIII began to close the monasteries in 1536 a number of monks who had received some training in surgery were cast adrift into the community. Men who had had practical experience in surgery in the army were also offering their services to the public. But by far the largest group of surgical practitioners was formed by the barbers, who were skilled in such minor procedures as blood-letting and tooth-extraction. The Company of Barbers was a well-established and prosperous body. In 1540 Thomas Vicary, the King's surgeon, succeeded in bringing about the union of the Company of Barbers with the Guild of Surgeons, to form the Company of Barber-Surgeons of the City of London. While the barbers gained in prestige, the surgeons hoped to use their increased strength and resources to establish lectures and regular demonstrations in anatomy.

Although they were only moderately successful in this regard, the surgeons became better educated, more prosperous, and more numerous until, two hundred years after the formation of the combined Company, they felt that the time had come to separate from the barbers. In 1745 the division occurred, with the establishment of the independent Company of Surgeons. One of the new Company's first acts was to decide on the construction of a Surgeons' Hall, with a lecture hall and facilities for carrying out anatomical demonstrations. The site chosen was near Newgate prison and the Old Bailey. William Cheselden, who became Master of the Company in 1746, drew up a plan for the lecture theatre and urged that it be the first part of the building to be constructed. However, because of delays to allow for alternative plans to be considered, the Company found that several other schools, notably that of William Hunter, had become so well established that the Company could not successfully compete against them. William's brother, John, the founder of scientific surgery and a great teacher, had built up a vast and unique collection of anatomical and pathological specimens. When John Hunter died in 1793 his collection was offered for sale to the British Government. But Britain was at war with France; Prime Minister William Pitt declined the offer, saying that he did not even have enough money to buy gunpowder! Hunter had died a poor man and the executors of his will had difficulty in making provision for his widow, but they did agree to continue the lease on the house in which the collection was stored. William Clift, a young man who had been Hunter's loyal assistant, continued to care for it as a labour of love. In 1799 the Government agreed to buy the collection for £15 000, a fraction of what it had cost Hunter. It was offered to the Royal College of Physicians, who declined it. The Corporation of Surgeons then agreed to be its custodians. The acquisition of such a collection was a step towards the achievement of the Corporation's aim of becoming a leading educational body.

In 1800 the Corporation received a new Charter and became the Royal College of Surgeons of London. To do justice to its enhanced status the College acquired land in Lincoln's Inn Fields, where its spacious new building was erected. Hunter's collection was moved to this site in 1812, and became the Hunterian Museum. The College rewarded Clift by appointing him Conservator of the Museum, to work under the direction of a five-member board of Curators.

In succeeding years specimens from other sources were added to the Museum in such numbers that in 1842 the College Council decided that the time had come for the whole collection to be reclassified and annotated. Edward Stanley of St Bartholomew's Hospital was asked by the Council to find a man to whom the work for the pathology section could be entrusted, and to supervise his labours. Stanley nominated James Paget. He knew that the latter's experience as Curator of the Hospital Museum would stand him in good stead. The appointment was an honour but, as with so many of Paget's commitments, the remuneration was small in proportion to the magnitude of the task. He gave up report-writing for the *Medical Gazette,* the least interesting of his journalist activities, so that he could spend at least two hours each day at the College. It was providential that his lodgings in Serle Street were only a stone's throw from Lincoln's Inn Fields.

Even this appointment was not awarded to Paget without some opposition being voiced. Richard Owen, who had shared with Paget the credit for discovering the *Trichina* parasite, was at first displeased at finding himself again competing with the younger man.

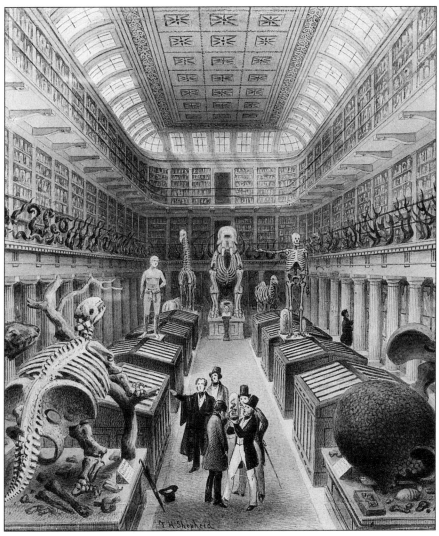

The Hunterian Museum, c1860. Water-colour by TH Shepherd. (Royal College of Surgeons).

In 1835 Owen had resigned from the lectureship in comparative anatomy at St Bartholomew's and had become William Clift's assistant at the Hunterian Museum. Clift retired in 1842 and Owen succeeded him as Conservator. In the event, it was Owen who compiled the new catalogue for the physiology section of the Museum, while Paget was responsible for the pathology section. The two men worked together in harmony for a number of years. When Owen resigned in 1856, in order to take up a senior appointment at the British Museum, he had established himself as an eminent zoologist and comparative anatomist. For Paget, too, the work for the Hunterian Museum led to better things.

A love of collections and collecting was a Paget trait. In later life James recalled with satisfaction his work on the Hunterian catalogue:

> ... It required a method of writing which is excellent for education in accuracy—an education terribly neglected. I described every specimen as I saw it standing or lying before me; nothing was to be told but what could be then and there seen; nothing that could be only imagined or remembered; there was to be mere translation from eyes to hand. And I venture to say that in tasks of scientific description no other method than this, where it is possible, should be trusted. Most artists know the contrast between a picture drawn from memory or imagination, and one from nature; so should scientific writers; nay, so should all writers, for oh! the lies, the controversies, the evil-speakings, the hindrances to truth that spring from the inaccuracies of those who believe themselves honest and well-meaning. Imprisonment with hard labour in catalogue-making might well befit them.[21]

Paget still deprived of operating experience

Circumstances thus continued to lead Paget into further study of pathology and away from practical surgery. While he was working on his writing and catalogue-making, one of his contemporaries was developing remarkable skills as an operator. William Fergusson, a Scot who had acquired his early surgical training in Edinburgh, was appointed Professor of Surgery at King's College Hospital, London, in 1840. In later years the skills of the two men appeared to their colleagues to be complementary—Fergusson the brilliant operator, Paget the astute diagnostician. In 1842, when Paget had yet to make his name, the exploits of Fergusson were attracting public attention. Thus, in a letter to George Paget written on 10 February, 1842, James refers to a report in *The Times* of an operation recently performed by Fergusson at King's College Hospital. The report read as follows:

Mr Fergusson, the principal surgeon of the King's College Hospital, performed yesterday, in the presence of nearly 200 medical students and a number of eminent physicians and surgeons, one of the most formidable surgical operations we ever witnessed in this country. The patient was a young girl, aged 12. She had a tumour of the size of an orange situated in a cavity in the upper jaw-bone. This morbid growth produced a hideous deformity of the face, as it extended into the nostrils and right orbit, pushing the eyeball nearly out of its socket. To remove this tumour Mr Fergusson had to take away half of the upper jaw-bone—the malar bone, on a portion of which the eye rests. In order to get at the tumour it was necessary in the first instance to make extensive incisions in the integuments of the face—in fact nearly the whole of the skin on one side of the cheek was dissected back, in order to expose the superior maxillary and malar bones. This was effected in less than a minute. The next step was to saw the bones, and remove them from their various detachments. Owing to the complicated structure of the parts, and the difficulty of getting the saw into its proper position, some little time elapsed before the tumour was removed; 16 minutes transpired before the tumour was extracted. The appearance of the patient after the bones were removed was truly awful. The whole of the face on the right side was laid bare, exposing the back part of the throat, tongue, and palate. The poor girl bore the operation with surprising fortitude; the pain she suffered must have been great. At the commencement she cried most piteously, but afterwards she exhibited great moral courage. In the performance of this dreadful operation Mr Fergusson evinced surprising coolness, great anatomical knowledge, and wonderful surgical dexterity. While all around him appeared dismayed at the nature of the operation, and turned pale at the frightful excisions which it was necessary to make, he (for we watched his face narrowly) never once lost his presence of mind. After the removal of the tumour the various portions of the skin were united together by sutures, and the poor girl was carried into the ward and placed in bed. We entertain sanguine hopes of the recovery of the girl, if she survives the shock given to the nervous system by the operation.[22]

The newspaper account portrays very clearly the horror of surgical operations before the advent of anaesthesia. The suffering of the patient, the strain on the surgeon who had to perform a difficult operation at lightning speed, and the presence of crowds of curious spectators in the operating theatre, were commonplace in 1842. Within Paget's lifetime surgical practice would be transformed, to the immeasurable benefit of humanity.

The first microscope arrives at St Bartholomew's
In 1842 the Hospital acquired its first microscope. At that time
there was very little work being done in Britain on the microscopic
appearance of normal and abnormal tissues. Paget saw this as an
opportunity to make a name for himself. He read all the published
articles on microscopy, added his own original material, and wrote
several extensive reviews of the subject. These were well received.
When the microscope arrived he was working on the first section of
his textbook of general anatomy. This section dealt with the skin
and its appendages, such as the nails, hair follicles, and sweat
glands; these were excellent topics for the microscopist. He therefore felt quite confident when, some months later, he submitted the
manuscript to Longmans, the publishers. A few days later it was
returned, with a note of refusal. After all his work this was at first
a bitter disappointment. The effort was not wasted, however. There
was consolation in being able to use the material in his lectures to
students.

As St Bartholomew's declines, Paget advances
Paget's increasing optimism about his future was linked, somewhat
paradoxically, with the observation that the fortunes of the
Hospital's medical school were continuing to decline. He explained
this in a letter to George, written at the beginning of the winter term
in October, 1842:

> I do not think there are more than half the number of new pupils
> that there were last year, and all is very dull. It is true that, on
> the whole, a small number of students have this year come to
> London, and some of the small Schools will probably be closed;
> but our deficiency is beyond all proportion greater than that of
> any other large School.

> This looks bad enough, for one whose bread depends on it: but I
> am not sure that it is really a bad thing for me. The school can
> never fall so low but that I should be profited by being a Lecturer;
> and it is quite clear now that if they wish to keep the school above
> water they must take in working men, and those of that small
> class of which I am senior. It is not easy to trace all the causes
> of this descent, but I believe, and have said plainly to some of the
> authorities, that the chief is in the anatomy department: there
> is, almost literally, no work done in the dissecting-rooms: after
> one o'clock, the dissecting rooms are absolutely empty.

> Affairs lately, I thank God, have seemed to be working towards
> a favourable change. Stanley told me a month ago that he,
> Lawrence, Burrows, and Roupell had decided to recommend to

the Governors that my demonstratorship should be advanced to a lectureship, and that my pupils should pay me. They propose to do this before next summer. But this was planned before the season opened: now, their favourable intentions *may* find a better field to place me in. Lawrence too, in the opening address (got up this year for the first time) took occasion to speak very highly of me—this occurring in the presence of the Treasurer and Almoners may do me much good when my name comes before them; at the last *émeute* I was hardly known to them, and suffered in consequence. On the whole, therefore, I cannot but hope that next October I shall be in a better position than I am now; and most assuredly for my comfort's sake I need be, for my work is more nearly incessant than ever.[23]

James had correctly judged the situation. Within a few months of his writing these observations the Governors embarked on an ambitious plan for the restoration of the medical school to its former status. The plan required the utilization of all the talented men available, without regard to their membership of the professional heirarchy.

In his memoirs Paget referred to the seven years that followed his admission to the Royal College of Surgeons as the 'waiting time'. It was a period of drudgery and disappointments, but it was also the period in which he matured, and in which he laid the foundations of the later years of fulfilment. The experiences of the waiting time strengthened those characteristics that were to set James Paget apart from lesser men.

Inclination and circumstances had combined to make him one of the new breed of surgeons, a scientist, rather than a virtuoso of the knife. He had already made several significant contributions to medical knowledge. He had discovered his talent for teaching and had made of this a secondary vocation that was both stimulating and satisfying. His relationship with his parents and the family at Yarmouth had matured. His love for them was as strong as ever, and would motivate him for years to come to make extraordinary sacrifices on their behalf. But he had established clearly that he was now living an independent life, and would make his own decisions on important personal matters. His engagement to Lydia North had withstood the test of years of waiting; both young people felt more certain than ever of the rightness of their choice. He had encountered for the first time the enmity of rivals, and had developed the perfect defence—tolerant understanding of his opponents, combined with strengthening of his own determination to succeed.

Chapter 5

The College Warden

In John Abernethy's hey-day, lectures at St Bartholomew's Hospital had regularly attracted audiences of several hundred, mostly students. In 1842 there were only thirty-six students enrolled for the winter term, the smallest number in the school's history. The medical committee acknowledged that it must appoint new teachers and improve the outmoded curriculum. The science of physiology was still relatively new, but it was advancing rapidly and no longer should be taught, as it was at St Bartholomew's, as a mere addendum to anatomy. Physiology was therefore deleted from the anatomy course, which was revised and renamed 'descriptive and surgical anatomy'. A new course of lectures, to be known as 'general anatomy and physiology' was introduced; the anatomy taught in this would be limited to the structural and functional relationships of organs.

At this juncture Edward Stanley, who had succeeded Abernethy as lecturer in anatomy, announced his resignation, so new lecturers had to be appointed for both courses. These events marked a turning point in James Paget's career. His classes in pathology had established his reputation as a teacher. It was well known that he had a special interest in general anatomy and had been writing a textbook on this subject. As a journalist on the staff of the *Quarterly Review* he had, for eight years, reported and reviewed recent advances in physiology, thereby acquiring a knowledge of this subject that none of his rivals could match. He seemed to be the logical choice for the lectureship in physiology. But past disappointments made him wary; he prepared his application with great care and steeled himself to face yet another setback. However, it seemed a good omen that Thomas Wormald chose this time to intimate that he wished to forget their past differences and to work cordially with Paget in the future.

Lectures in general anatomy and physiology
On 30 May, 1843, it was announced that James Paget was to be the lecturer in general anatomy and physiology. Samuel Paget wrote to James, expressing the family's joy and their bright hopes for his future. Mrs Paget was now so severely disabled that she could add only a scrawled footnote to her husband's letter: 'I say Amen to the above.'

The appointment of the lecturer in descriptive and surgical anatomy caused much more controversy. The two chief contenders were

Thomas Wormald and Frederick Skey. Skey, the more senior, was an assistant surgeon at the Hospital and also lectured at the Aldersgate Street school. Some fourteen years previously Skey and Wormald had competed for the Hospital's demonstratorship in anatomy. Although Wormald had had the support of Abernethy, Skey was the successful candidate. Four years later Skey resigned from the demonstratorship in order to teach at the neighbouring Aldersgate Street school. There he had attracted large and appreciative audiences, at a time when the Hospital school was declining. Wormald meanwhile had become demonstrator in anatomy and also assistant surgeon at the Hospital. As on the first occasion, each of the two men had his group of supporters in the Hospital; once again it was Skey who triumphed. Paget summed up his feelings about the man who was to be his colleague:

> It was a good thing, in every way, that Skey was brought from the rival school. He was one of the Assistant-Surgeons of the Hospital; and peace was hardly possible while he was in open competition with his colleagues. Besides, he was at least as good a teacher as Wormald, and he was popular with many, and not very difficult to deal with—a warm-hearted, impetuous, generous, and careless man. His anatomy was of the older sort, and he had not time even if he had inclination to modernize it: for his ambition and necessity combined to make him very anxious for surgical practice. We worked pretty well together, and though we seldom quite agreed we never quarrelled.[1]

A new college for the students

Meanwhile the Hospital Governors contemplated another important development at the school. They realized the need to improve facilities for students and also to provide these immature young men with some form of supervision. There were similar problems at other London hospitals. The Revd Mr North, James's future brother-in-law, had tried to persuade the Governors of St George's Hospital to establish a students' residence which, in some respects, would resemble a university college. The students would be required to attend morning chapel and would dine formally with the Warden and guests each evening. The Warden would see that rules of conduct were strictly observed within the college; he would also act as adviser to students with academic or personal problems.

Mr North's suggestion was not adopted at St George's, but the discussion it engendered spread to other hospitals. At St Bartholomew's several of the medical men, James Paget among them, realized the merit of the proposal and succeeded in winning the support of the Hospital's treasurer, James Bentley. Paget found much to admire in Bentley:

He was a truly admirable man; an example of that admirable class, the rich merchants given to good works; men who make money with great care, and give it away with as great liberality; men who are exact and orderly in business; sometimes even exacting, when those they deal with are not needy; winning money as keenly as others would win games at cards; counting their money as the fairest estimate of their success in a difficult and honest competition; but, once counted, giving it freely, and with it giving their time and strong will and knowledge to the management of great charities. There were, as there still are, several of the kind among the Governors of St Bartholomew's; and Mr Bentley was the best among them: rich and still making money as much as if he wanted it for himself, generous, pious, rigid, requiring everyone's whole duty to be done, resolute for everything that he thought right. Under his rule some of the greatest improvements in the buildings and arrangements of the Hospital were made. The earnestness which he showed in the endeavour to make them, even at great expense, as good as possible, was a novelty at that time: it has been nearly habitual ever since.[2]

James Bentley formed a college committee of enthusiastic and able men. They soon decided on the site of the college—a row of rather shabby houses in the adjacent Duke Street. Six of the houses were renovated and furnished, another was demolished to make way for the building of a kitchen and dining hall. Caterers were appointed and estimates of the cost of conducting the college were

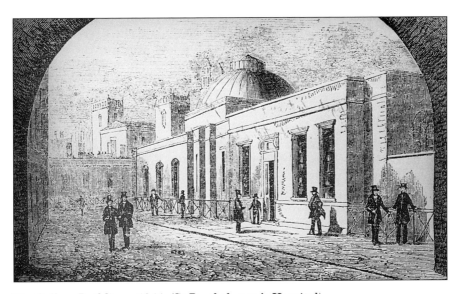

The College Buildings, 1844. (St Bartholomew's Hospital).

approved. By mid-1843 the College of St Bartholomew's Hospital
was close to becoming a reality. It was time to appoint the first
Warden. Paget's support for the project, and his interest in the
welfare of students, were well known; the committee had frequently
called on his help during the planning period. On 8 August, 1843,
the appointment was offered to him and he accepted it.

Paget as Warden
These two successes in less than three months gave Paget fresh
heart. They justified his decision to centre all his hopes on St
Bartholomew's Hospital. Furthermore, they had been achieved
without any of the bitter rivalry that accompanied his previous,
unsuccessful applications. Although his salary as Warden would be
only £50 per annum, he would live in College and thus save the cost
of board and lodgings. He would receive payment for his physiology
lectures, in addition to his Warden's salary. His professional and
financial prospects were so much improved that it was now possible
to fix a date for his marriage. James and Lydia decided that it would
take place in the summer of 1844.

Before taking up his duties as Warden James visited the family
in Yarmouth. His mother's health was deteriorating and Charles
was also seriously ill. His two sisters, Patty and Kate, nursed the
invalids and kept house for their father and brothers. The brewery
continued to lose money and even Samuel Paget had at last
accepted that its sale was inevitable. James's pleasure in his own
success was largely overshadowed by concern for the family.

After spending a month at Yarmouth he returned to his lodgings
at Serle Street for the last time; on 28 September, 1843, he moved
into the College and began a new life. For years he had lived such
a solitary existence that while he worked late at night the sound of
a footstep on the stairs was a rare and startling event. Now he
presided over an establishment of twenty-three lively young men.
Whereas previously he had usually taken his evening meal by
himself 'in some cheap chop-house', he now dined in College,
enjoying good food and congenial company.

His duties as Warden and his commitment to the preparation
and delivery of six lectures per week made heavy demands on his
time. He had almost ceased to be a medical journalist, retaining
only the association he enjoyed the most, the one with the *Quarterly
Review*. Now this also had to be relinquished, but he was happy to
find that his friendship with John Forbes and Sir James Clark
continued.

After his first week as Warden James wrote to Lydia of his hopes
for the College's future:

I begin now to believe that it may be permanently beneficial, and to hope that I am the husbandman of a seed which in years will produce an abundant harvest of good to men, and of acceptable service to God. The students seem well disposed to conformity both with the rules and with good manners; and if, after the habit of a week or two in this, I can only persuade them to work, the scheme with God's help is safe. But in nothing have I ever felt so thoroughly my own inefficiency as in this part of my duties.[3]

A month later he was again writing of his difficulty in convincing the students of the value of hard work and early rising:

... All matters here work-on steadily. And when I speak of difficulties arising in the management of the College, these are only such as must arise in a society of 24 men of the most diverse dispositions, and many of them with the most obscure notions of the purpose of the place in which they find themselves. I begin to find that, like Judge Jeffreys, I have a rough side to my tongue, which I can now work almost as easily as the smooth one. I have succeeded I trust in reproof—*rowing* in good earnest, till a culprit even wept. But don't talk of these things: and I find (thank God) that the burden of them grows each day, by habit, easier.

So do *not* the lectures. I did wrongly to start so vigorously; for now I must try to maintain the same pace; and I am terribly put to it, to excuse all that is dry. However, happily, the congregation continues large. That at morning prayers is less steady—the men give no worse excuse than that it is hard to get up so early, and this will be difficult to correct, especially as I think it much better than any *conscientious* excuse against Church services. I am glad to say that I do not think there is a *strictly conscientious* man in the College: they are all therefore nearly manageable.[4]

More family bereavements
On 22 November, 1843, the family suffered the shock of the death of their mother. For six years they had known that she had a progressive and incurable complaint, but her courage had deceived them into believing her condition to be less grave than it was. Her son Alfred wrote of her:

If there were one thing that would tell the history of the house it would be my mother's handwriting from first to last: the bold tall characters of the early specimens, and the shaking defiant effort against nerves that marks the later ones, and asks me 'to excuse a steel pen.' I wish I could but for a moment recall any one of those single words with which she would deliver an opinion on the white slate, as if she gloried in having left her spirit among some and all of her children—how she would mock at her own infirmity of hand. A single word would display the wit, the pungent sarcasm, the daring high spirit that the heavy calamity of her illness had dumbed but left untamed within. Think of her strange mixture of generosity to the weak and defiance to the strong . . .[5]

Only a few days after his mother's death James received an honour that would have given her great pleasure. He was one of the three hundred foundation Fellows elected by the Council of the Royal College of Surgeons. The list of Fellows included many distinguished names and James Paget was one of the youngest.

In March of the following year the family suffered another bereavement. Charles, who had been fighting a losing battle against sickness and depression for many years, at last succumbed. Alfred wrote of him:

Until the last years of his life, when melancholia overcame him, Charles's quick eye and ready pencil had constantly recorded, in delightful sketches, the little episodes of family life in which Frank especially revelled. Many of them still exist, miniature paintings, caricatures from the window of passers by or local celebrities, finely detailed painting of his insect collections, showing a rare and versatile skill. Almost all his life he had been an invalid, but he had not fallen behind his brothers, in a family which was wholehearted in all its undertakings. His death threw upon Frank more work and greater responsibility, but it brought him more than ever into companionship with his father.[6]

Although there was now only Frank to help him at the brewery, Samuel Paget still tried to postpone its sale. A railway line that was being built between Norwich and Yarmouth would terminate close to the brewery; he hoped that the land would greatly increase in value, if only he could wait long enough.

Paget marries
On 23 May, 1844, James and Lydia were quietly married, after an engagement of nearly eight years. The ceremony took place in London, at St Mary's Church, Bryanston Square. A day's visit to Oxford was as much honeymoon as they could afford, before they returned to rooms in the College. A few weeks later they were able to move into the house that the Hospital had acquired as a residence for the Warden. The marriage that began with so little outward show was to last for over fifty years, unmarred by any serious disagreement or faltering of affection. In 1846 their first child, a

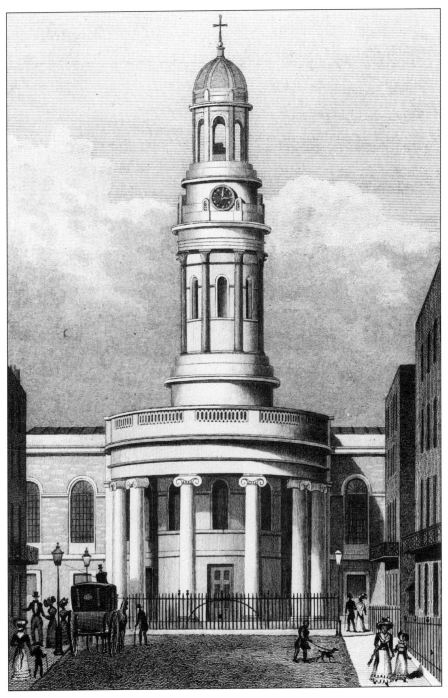

St Mary's Church, Bryanston Square. (Guildhall Library, London).

daughter whom they named Catherine, was born. In old age James recalled how easily he was able to make the transition from bachelorhood to married life. Instead of distracting him, his new contentment enabled him to work with even greater enthusiasm:

> From this time, the 'being alone' was the being alone with one who never failed in love, in wise counsel, in prudence and in gentle care of me. With her it was easy to work and be undisturbed by anything going-on around me; a habit which I can advise every one to learn. Her admirable music and her singing, with a matchless gentle voice and a pure cultivated style, were a refreshing accompaniment to my evening reading and writing; and when these were over, she wrote for me, copying for the press my roughly written manuscripts, sitting with me till midnight or far into the morning, all alone, or, after a time, with the baby brought down in its cradle and watched and fed.

> I can recommend the plan to all young married people. It is an intensely happy one and may teach them to be able to work in the midst of what are commonly called interruptions. I owe to it that I have never once needed to leave my family or any tolerably quiet party of friends in order to work alone or undisturbed; whether for writing, reading, or any other similar work, no kind of good music or talking has ever interrupted me: I have thoroughly enjoyed them even while at work.[7]

Lydia Paget supported her husband's efforts to counsel students who were in trouble, by making them feel they were always welcome to visit the Warden's house. On Sunday evenings those students who remained in College were invited to enjoy music and supper with the Warden and his wife. This informal hospitality became a custom that James and Lydia continued long after he had ceased to be Warden of the College. Their friends knew that on Sunday evenings the Pagets welcomed all who cared to join them for music, conversation, and refreshments.

The brewery is sold

In February, 1845, the brewery was at last sold. The building did not remain as a reminder of the good times that had passed, for shortly after the sale it was demolished and its bricks used to build the foundations of a Catholic church in Yarmouth. Frank had to find new employment. George and James made inquiries on his behalf and he himself followed a number of leads without success. Then, in May, he learned of a vacancy for a customs officer at Liverpool. Several weeks of interviews and examinations were followed by a course of instruction; then he was ready to take up his duties in September. The family arranged that Patty and Kate would take turns in staying with Frank at Liverpool, to keep house for him.

A historical record of William Harvey
There were other notable events in that year. James had somehow found time to compile a record of all the references to William Harvey in the Hospital archives; to these he added historical and biographical notes. The essay, of thirty-seven pages, was published by John Churchill under the title *Records of Harvey, In Extracts from the Journals of the Royal Hospital of St Bartholomew.*

Harvey was appointed physician to the Hospital in 1609, when he was thirty-one years old. He had already formulated his theory of the function of the heart and the blood vessels, but he waited nearly twenty years before publishing his historic treatise *On the Motion of the Heart and Blood in Animals.* Harvey was also keenly interested in the administration of the Hospital; in 1615 he drew up a list of sixteen regulations for approval by the Governors. Paget reproduced the regulations and added his own explanatory notes and comments. Harvey's third regulation stated:

> That all such as are c'tefied by the do^r uncurable & scandelous or infeccous shalbe putt out of the said howse, or to be sent to an out-howse; And in case of suddaine inconvenience this to be done by the do^r or apothecary.[8]

Paget clarified this cryptic instruction by outlining the history of the Hospital's satellite institutions. Between the twelfth and fifteenth centuries, when leprosy was endemic in London, people afflicted with this disease were segregated in small outlying hospitals, called the Locks. Two of the Locks were administered by the Governors of St Bartholomew's Hospital; one, at Southwark, was for men; the other, at Kingsland, was for women. By the sixteenth century leprosy had practically disappeared, but syphilis had taken its place as a severe and widespread infectious disease. It was the policy of the Hospital to send to the Locks patients suffering from syphilis and also patients with incurable diseases of other kinds. This rule had not been rigidly enforced, and at the time that Harvey wrote his instruction patients in both these categories were being admitted to the wards of the Hospital in large numbers. The Locks disappeared when the Hospital was rebuilt in the eighteenth century, special wards then being set aside for the treatment of syphilis.

In another of his regulations Harvey stipulated that the Hospital's surgeon (John Woodall) would always seek the opinion of the physician in difficult cases, that only the physician could prescribe medicines to be taken internally, and that the surgeon would 'in a decent & orderly manner p'ceed by the do^rs dir-reccons . . .' Much as he admired Harvey, Paget was too much the surgeon to allow a physician's claims to supremacy to pass unchallenged. Thus he wrote:

> The prohibition of the surgeons from the prescribing of inward physick, even in surgical cases, was so fully supported by the law, as put in force at the frequent instance of the College of Physicians in Harvey's time, that it would have been vain for the surgeons to protest against it. . . . Twice in Harvey's time the surgeons made attempts to obtain from Parliament and the King the right to give what they deemed good to help their external applications; pleading very truly 'the great and heavy burthen to the Common-wealth in general, when for every hurt apperteyning to the Chirurgion's cure the Patient must be forced to entertain a Surgeon, a Physician, and an Apothecary;' but all in vain. The College of Physicians was then nearly as irresistible in the execution, as it was inflexible in the assertion, of its rights.[9]

Harvey also believed that the physician should maintain secrecy about the remedies he used, but that 'every chirurgeon shall shewe & declare unto the Do^r . . . what he findeth, & what he useth to every externall malady'. Paget, living in more enlightened times, could not condone the efforts of either physicians or surgeons to be secretive about their treatments:

> We cannot wonder at the surgeons protesting at the inequality of the rules which secured secrecy for the physicians' prescriptions, and publicity for theirs. I cannot find how the protest was disposed of; but the probability is, that the surgeons were, as usual in those days, put down.

> It is not a little strange to find Harvey, who was not more esteemed for his science than for the stedfastness and devotion with which he maintained the dignity of his order, adopting a practice which is now characteristic of quackery. The custom of his time made that honest which is now, more justly, shameful. In none of the many prosecutions of empirics by the College of Physicians, recorded in Dr Goodall's history, is the secrecy of their modes of practice mentioned as an aggravation of their offences; nor is it, I think, in any considerable work of that period, regarded as a custom of questionable propriety. Indeed, it would be difficult to find better evidence that the custom of secrecy in practice was both usual and reputable than these rules afford, in which we find Harvey, the high-minded defender and benefactor

of the College of Physicians, demanding it for himself, and the surgeons of the hospital, of whom two at least were 'Masters in Surgery', protesting against the proposal to make their secrets known.[10]

Later in the same year Paget completed another notable work. His catalogue of the Hospital museum, begun in 1837, was published in October, 1846, under the title *A Descriptive Catalogue of the Anatomical Museum of St Bartholomew's Hospital.* As well as listing over two thousand specimens, it contained notes and references designed to make it a valuable aid to students of pathology.

Arris and Gale Professorship
The year 1847 began auspiciously with his election to the Arris and Gale Professorship of the Royal College of Surgeons. The holder of this appointment was required to deliver six lectures over a period of two weeks, on a subject of his own choosing. Paget, at the age of thirty-six, was unusually young to have been awarded this honour. He knew that he would have a critical audience and that his performance would significantly affect his professional reputation.

The subject he chose was Nutrition; by this he meant not only the nutrition of the body as a whole, but also the regulation of the supply of nutrients to the various tissues under normal and abnormal conditions. In his letters to George he reported the progress of the lectures:

May 6th.—I have given two of my College Lectures. They were well received, the theatre was crowded, and those whom I can trust to tell the truth have praised them; so I hope to be re-elected Professor. My father was at the first, and enjoyed the circumstances immensely.

May 19th.—My lectures are over, and thank God well over— their reception was most gratifying, and I have been assured from all quarters that they were well thought of. They will be printed shortly in the 'Medical Gazette.'[11]

His re-election to the Arris and Gale Professorship each year for the next five years was proof that they continued to be 'well thought of' by his peers. His subjects for the six years were:

1847—Nutrition; 1848—The Life of the Blood; 1849—The Processes of Repair and Reproduction after Injuries; 1850—Inflammation; 1851—Tumours; and 1852—Malignant Tumours.

Paget believed that it was his work for the College Museum,

particularly in the conservation of Hunter's specimens, that had caused him to be elected in 1847. For this reason he thought it appropriate to base the lectures on the material in the Museum:

> As circumstances had decided the subject, it seemed well to let them determine, also, the method, and to adopt that which was most natural to one engaged in the simultaneous practice of surgery and teaching of physiology. Thus guided, I designed to give lectures which might illustrate the general pathology of the principal surgical diseases, in conformity with the larger and more exact doctrines of physiology; and the plan seemed the more reasonable, because it was in accordance with the constant design of the great founder of the Museum.[12]

Before he gave the first series his ability as a speaker was known only to those who had attended his physiology classes at St Bartholomew's Hospital. As the Arris and Gale Professor he addressed large and discerning audiences; the theatre at the Royal College of Surgeons was filled to capacity for each of his lectures, and among those who heard him were many of the nation's leading surgeons. His application of recent advances in physiology and pathology to the practice of surgery caught their interest, while his skilful presentation made the lectures a pleasurable experience. The Arris and Gale lectures established James Paget's reputation as a public speaker of outstanding ability.

In later life he advised ambitious young medical men not to underestimate the importance to their careers of the ability to speak well in public, although he also cautioned them against appearing too eager to rush to the rostrum. Whenever they did speak they should be well prepared, with material carefully selected and a suitable style of delivery perfected by practice. His own style may well have been modelled on that of his old teacher, William Lawrence. Paget's voice was not strong or resonant; he spoke quietly, but very clearly, using the simple English favoured by masters of the language. He did not use dramatic gestures or inflections of the voice. Every lecture was so carefully prepared that he could deliver it without referring to his notes, unless quoting another authority. But the effect he had on his audiences cannot be explained by considering only these attributes of style. Great orators are able to convey their feelings, as well as their ideas, so that for each member of the audience the occasion is a memorable experience. Paget's contemporaries leave us in no doubt that he had this gift.

Paget elected Assistant Surgeon
In February, 1847, he arrived at an important milestone in his

career; he was elected Assistant Surgeon to St Bartholomew's Hospital. Nine years previously he had made a token application, knowing that he had no chance of succeeding. In the intervening years his standing at the Hospital had so much improved that he entered this contest quietly confident of the outcome, even though his two opponents were both former apprentices of Edward Stanley. William Pennington, a pleasant, but not highly ambitious man, was a candidate mainly because his family expected it of him. Andrew McWhinnie, on the other hand, was desperately eager for the appointment. Dr Horace Dobell, who was a student at the Hospital in 1847, later recalled an incident associated with this election:

> I was witness to a battle-royal between Mr Paget and Mr McWhinnie. McWhinnie was his senior in age and standing at the Hospital, and had waited wearily for a vacancy in the Assistant-Surgeonship. Paget was waiting too, and had done such work as to have richly earned promotion, and he had set his life-prospects on getting this post. McWhinnie thought he ought not to be opposed by a junior, and learning that Paget meant to 'put up', he tackled him one day in the Museum, where I happened to be working. First he tried persuasion, then threats of defeat. Paget kept calm but obstinately asserting that he intended to stand. McWhinnie grew hotter and hotter, and they retired into the Curator's little room to fight it out. The storm grew on both sides—but the younger man never budged an inch from his first position, that he meant to put up, and meant to fight hard, and meant to win.[13]

The appointment was of great practical value to Paget because it allowed him to remedy the defect in his training that had troubled him since his student days. As an assistant surgeon he had ample opportunity to gain experience in operative and clinical surgery; the fact that he lived at the Hospital and was readily available in emergencies brought him additional surgical cases. On some days he saw as many as two hundred patients.

The introduction of anaesthesia
Paget was fortunate in that his appointment almost coincided with an event that transformed surgical practice—the introduction of anaesthesia. James Young Simpson read his historic paper on the use of ether at a meeting of the Royal Medical Society of Edinburgh, in March, 1847. Ether at once came into use at St Bartholomew's Hospital, but mainly for dental extractions. When Simpson read a second paper in November, in which he described the advantages of chloroform over ether, anaesthesia for surgical operations gained acceptance and was soon used routinely. By 1850 over seven

thousand anaesthetics had been administered at St Bartholomew's Hospital. Thus it was only for a period of less than a year after his appointment as assistant surgeon that Paget was subjected to the stress of operating on conscious patients. Lydia Paget is said to have welcomed the innovation with enthusiasm equal to her husband's. The Warden's house was within earshot of the Hospital's operating theatre; the happiness of her first few years of residence there had been marred by the inescapable sounds of anguish that emanated from the theatre on operating days.

The use of the microscope
Work in the post-mortem room of the Hospital occupied much of Paget's time since his appointment as Curator of the museum. John Hunter would have approved his diligent efforts to relate the findings after death with what had been known or surmised about the living patient, since this is probably the most effective single means of improving medical knowledge. Paget had begun to make use of the microscope as soon as the Hospital acquired one in 1842. Now he was using it not only to examine the finer structure of his post-mortem specimens, but also as an experimental tool. He repeated many of the basic experiments in physiology described by pioneers in this field and devised new ones to widen his knowledge of the body's response to disease and injury. His letters to his brother George at this time abound in requests for supplies of experimental animals such as tadpoles, newts, and bats, creatures that were not readily available in large numbers in the city. The fruits of all this work enriched his lectures at the Hospital and at the Royal College of Surgeons. In 1848 his name appeared in print as that of co-author, with William Kirkes, of the *Handbook of Physiology*. Kirkes had attended Paget's lectures as a student and was instrumental in having them published in textbook form. The book was well received and went through several editions.

Changes in family life
On 9 March, 1848, their first son was born to Lydia and James. By happy coincidence the birth date was the anniversary of the day in 1830 when James's apprenticeship deed with Charles Costerton was signed. The child was christened John Rahere, the name possibly reflecting James's hope that his son was also destined to be a medical man at St Bartholomew's Hospital.

An objective observer of the young Paget family would have said that James and Lydia were poor and that James was overworked. But being constantly short of money did not seriously mar their happiness and James, although often very tired, derived great pleasure from his work. Neither of them minded that on the rare occasion that they accepted an invitation to dinner, they had to walk home in order to save the cab fare. Their needs were modest. They enjoyed the company of a few good friends at the Hospital, and were content with such simple entertainment as a stroll in the Hospital Square on a summer evening.

The only dark shadow over James's existence at this time was the worsening plight of the family at Yarmouth. A few months previously his father had been forced to sell some of his paintings; the proceeds of the sale had quickly disappeared in the payment of debts. Samuel Paget had to bring himself to sell more of the family's possessions and move into a smaller house. An auction sale of the contents of the house on the Quay was to be held in October, 1848.

Patty was at Liverpool looking after Frank; the task of organizing the sale fell to Kate, since even to talk of it distressed her father. It was Kate who instructed the auctioneer, Mr Pettingill, and made the difficult decisions about which items were to be kept. On the eve of the auction, when everything that was for sale had been numbered and put on display, she carefully collected and locked away the few possessions the family would keep. Then her pride dictated that the whole house must be dusted and polished, so that curious intruders could find nothing to criticize.

Poor Kate's industry went unrewarded. The sale next day was a disaster. Furniture, pictures, books, and silver, all of them treasured mementoes of members of the family, were sold for a fraction of their worth. When the crowd departed Kate wrote to Alfred:

As I took the candle and walked across the poor soiled vestibule and went into the Library to see the remains of the once pretty books, and saw my Shakespeare shelf half empty, I did feel a more bitter pang than I thought I could. So bad was it, that at one time Mr Pettingill had some idea of stopping the sale altogether . . .

I can never I think, pass more bitter hours than I have lately— to feel, as I have, my mother's pride rise, and bitter sorrow that people who in her lifetime never would have entered this darling house have come and picked and carried away our beauties at a ruinous loss. But take comfort to yourself. I have got under lock and key the darlings of the whole House. My mother's memory shall not be profaned by the people's scorn of the things; so before they shall have them I will smash and destroy them all; let us go to ruin with the broken fragments, rather than take the few paltry pence we should get for them: this is a bad feeling; but I am sore, very sore just now.[14]

But Kate managed to throw off her depression. 'After all', she had written to Alfred before the sale, 'happiness does not live in a silver dish'. When, as Christmas approached, James suggested that they should hold a last family celebration in the old home, she gave the idea her support. George was at first sceptical that they could make it a happy occasion, but he was soon won over and James, George, and Alfred agreed that they would each take with them a contribution to the traditional Christmas feast. Frank and Patty

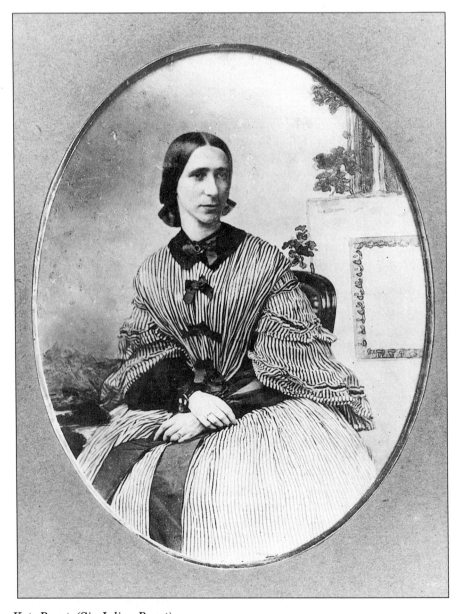

Kate Paget. (Sir Julian Paget).

would come home from Liverpool. But the celebration was not to be. Frank's health had been declining for several months, and in the last few weeks he had had to take leave of absence from his work. He was well enough to journey home to Yarmouth early in December, but nine days before Christmas he rapidly became much worse, and within a few hours he was dead.

Frank's previous absence from home did not lessen the blow. He had been a faithful correspondent and, although his letters told of his declining health, they were always so good-humoured and optimistic that it was hard to accept that his life had suddenly ended. Alfred wrote:

> They are leaving the house where, since it was built, my Mother, Arthur and Charles and Frank, besides all those sisters and brothers whom I never knew, have died. And the shutters will be closed for ever. Oh, what life and activity in every room of that house and not least in Frank's. For he used his whole life, his worldly means, his time, his money, his society, but as an instrument of some higher power. And he made a joke of it all.[15]

On 14 February Samuel Paget and his two daughters moved into a small house in St George's Terrace, Yarmouth, taking with them just enough of their possessions to make the new home comfortable and inviting. Kate and Patty worked all day; then, just as everything was in place and dusk was falling, they realized that it was St Valentine's Day, the day that the family had always celebrated. Kate dispatched her father to the old home to collect any parcels that had been left for them, and then she herself hurried out to buy a special cake for supper. Later that evening Kate wrote to Alfred, describing how, after the turmoil of the move, they had honoured St Valentine as the family had in the past:

> Oh, how many recollections crowded on me, the many years ago when I used to go out . . . to leave the Valentines! I felt as if the spirits of those dear ones, who have been taken to that blessed rest they could not find here, moved around me at each act I did today. Think me crazy or romantic, you will forgive these wild ideas. Dearest Mama and dear, dear Frank would have been pleased that Papa should not be forgotten and the *14th Cake* was there![16]

A month later the members of the Shipping Clubs of Yarmouth voted Mr Paget a small pension. He was grateful for the income, but even more pleased by this demonstration of affection and esteem by his old colleagues. The pension eased only slightly Samuel Paget's pressing financial problems. The house on the Quay had been heavily mortgaged and he owed large sums to business creditors. George, James, and Alfred entered into an agreement to help support their father and sisters, and to pay off all his debts, even if it took them many years. James acknowledged that some people would think it strange that the brothers signed a legal document to this effect; he commented, 'Business never hinders love: mere understandings often do.' The burden they were assuming was formidable—'a terrible sum to look at, but not to be evaded: it has great value for the suppression of many projects I might otherwise be tempted to indulge in.'

Paget's career continues to develop

As he faced this new task James had the satisfaction of seeing another completed. The catalogue of the Museum of the Royal College of Surgeons was finished in May, 1849, after seven years' work. Its five volumes contained notes on 3520 specimens, more than twice the number listed in William Clift's catalogue of 1830. The preface gives some indication of how carefully Paget had striven to preserve the Hunterian tradition, while introducing advances in knowledge that occurred in the half-century since Hunter's death:

> In arranging the collection and preparing the Catalogue, every specimen was repeatedly examined by Mr Stanley and Mr Paget. The descriptions of what the preparations still display to the naked eye were written by Mr Paget, and, after revision and comparison with the specimens, were sanctioned by Mr Stanley. These gentlemen are, therefore, jointly responsible for the correctness of the descriptions. In the case of the Hunterian specimens, Mr Paget has inserted, in every possible instance, the histories or other detailed notices concerning them; employing and verifying for this purpose the numerous references which had been already made by Mr Clift to the manuscripts and published writings of Mr Hunter. He has also given all the details respecting the other preparations that could be collected from oral and manuscript communications, from contemporary publications and from other sources.[17]

As well as completing the catalogue he had given his third series of Arris and Gale lectures. The subject for this year was the processes of repair after injury, and again the lectures had been very enthusiastically received. Despite all this academic activity he continued to make the most of his opportunities to operate. In January, 1849, he noted on a letter to George, 'I did a formidable operation on Saturday . . . Thank God I got well through it, and the patient is making good progress: but it was one of the hardest cases of tumour I have seen meddled with.' Two months later he was able to report his first lithotomy (the operation for the removal of a stone from the bladder), 'I performed my first lithotomy on Saturday—slowly and not, perhaps, too dexterously—but not confusedly—and, as I hope, very safely, for the boy is doing well.' With his duties as Warden, in addition to his lectures and operating, Paget was working harder than ever. He had to decline George's invitation to join him on a short holiday:

> I should thoroughly enjoy a holiday with you, and I would take one if it were not so expensive—not of money, but in subsequent work. The time I have to give to my College Lectures is taken so completely from what should be given to other duties that, while they go on, all other things fall into arrear. I reckon that for every holiday I must do more than a day's work, and that therefore the least work will need to be done if I take no whole holidays till near the close of the summer. Then (D.V.) I hope we may get to Yarmouth; but till then I am resolved to work on gently and take occasional half-holidays and good nights' rests. Not that I feel the need of these luxuries—but I begin to think I cannot be so unlike other people as to be able to endure much longer what others soon fail under.[18]

Cholera epidemic in London
When he was an apprentice in Yarmouth Paget had observed the cholera epidemic of 1831. In the summer of 1849 another outbreak of the disease occurred, with heavy loss of life in London. Previously none of the London hospitals would admit cholera patients to their wards, for fear that the disease would spread to other patients, but in the epidemic of 1849 St Bartholomew's allocated two wards, Bentley and Lucas, to the care of cholera victims. During the four months that the epidemic lasted, 478 cases were admitted to the Hospital, and of these 199 died. One of those who died was a member of the Hospital staff.

Paget, as a surgeon, was not directly involved with the treatment of cholera patients, but he read with interest the letters and articles in the medical journals in which various theories as to the nature of the disease were advanced. He was unconvinced by the arguments that a fungus was responsible. He probably did not then know of the work of Dr John Snow, who studied the distribution of cases in the most severely affected areas of the city, and thereby gained a valuable insight into the nature of the epidemic. In 1838 Snow had begun his professional life as a general practitioner, but nine years later he was attracted to the new field of anaesthesia. He was shocked to see how carelessly ether was being administered by men who knew nothing of its dangers. With characteristic thoroughness he studied the properties of ether, and later of chloroform, and soon won a reputation as the first specialist anaesthetist. His services were much in demand by London's leading surgeons. Nevertheless, when the epidemic of cholera struck in 1849 he found time to record detailed observations on the spread of the epidemic. He began to suspect that the disease could be acquired by drinking water that had been contaminated with sewage. London's water supply was then in the hands of a number of private companies, some of which obtained their water from sites in the Thames adjacent to sewage effluents. Snow suggested that when this sewage contained excreta from cholera victims the water supply became contaminated with the cholera 'poison'. In 1849 he published a pamphlet entitled *The Mode of Communication of Cholera*. This provoked considerable interest at the time, but as the epidemic waned the medical profession and the general public lost interest in the subject. Snow again devoted his energies to his anaesthetic practice. On 7 April 1853 he was called upon to administer chloroform to the Queen during the birth of Prince Leopold; the publicity given to this event helped to overcome prejudice against the use of anaesthesia during childbirth. Nevertheless, he did not lose his interest in the epidemiology of cholera and another epidemic was soon to give him the opportunity to perform even more significant work on this subject.

Paget's reputation as a lecturer contributes to the renewed success of St Bartholomew's Hospital

As the decade reached its close the Hospital medical school was seen to be thriving. The number of students enrolled for the winter term of 1849–50 exceeded one hundred and fifty, and the College had been enlarged so that it could accommodate thirty-two men. This success was partly due to the reforms introduced in 1843, but it also owed much to the growing reputation of James Paget as a lecturer. Whereas Abernethy had informed and entertained his students, Paget inspired them to revere their profession. An article that appeared in the *St Bartholomew's Hospital Reports* for 1859 was written as a tribute to another surgeon, Sir William Savory, but it contains a brief reference to James Paget that shows how profoundly Paget impressed his students:

> It was at the commencement of the winter-session in October, 1846, that I first saw William Savory: the place, the dissecting-room of St Bartholomew's; the time, soon after nine in the morning, when the early refreshment of Paget's lecture at eight had ended, and his audience dispersing broke the deep silence that had held them listening spell-bound to the words of the master of surgical pathology during the previous hour.[19]

Visit by Dr Elizabeth Blackwell

It was Paget's reputation that attracted to St Bartholomew's the first woman doctor to be seen in London. Elizabeth Blackwell was born in Bristol in 1821. Her family migrated to America when she was eleven years old, and she grew up in New York State. Her ambition to study medicine was at first thwarted by the refusal of the leading medical schools of New York and Pennsylvania to accept a woman as a student. Eventually she gained entry to a school at Geneva, NY, and graduated MD in 1849. Dr Blackwell decided to continue her medical studies in Europe, but again met with hostility. When she eventually obtained a post at La Maternite, the famous lying-in hospital in Paris, it was only as a student midwife. Once, while syringing the infected eyes of a newborn, she accidently splashed pus from the infant into one of her own eyes. This led to a severe infection that destroyed the sight of her left eye; some months later she had to have the eye removed and replaced with a glass eye. It was during this illness that she learned that she had been granted permission to continue her studies at St Bartholomew's Hospital, a cousin in England having approached Mr Paget on her behalf. Paget obtained the approval of the Hospital's House Committee and then sent her a cordial letter of welcome. By October she was well enough to travel to London for the beginning of the winter term of 1850. She wrote to her family in America:

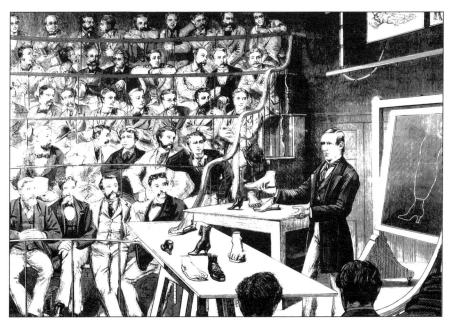

Paget Lecturing to Students at St Bartholomew's Hospital. (St Bartholomew's Hospital).

My first introduction to St Bartholomew's was at a breakfast at Mr Paget's. He has a house within the hospital boundaries, and a special oversight of the students. At the commencement of each session he invites the students to breakfast in parties of about a dozen and to one of those breakfasts I, on my arrival, was invited. The students seemed to be gentlemanly fellows, and looked with

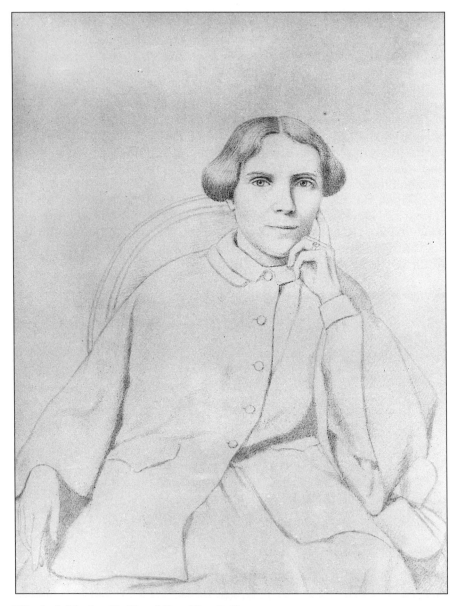

Elizabeth Blackwell. (Royal Free Hospital).

some curiosity at their new companion; the conversation was general and pleasant, the table well covered; Mrs Paget very sensible and agreeable, so that it was quite a satisfactory time.[20]

Before she made her first appearance at the pathology lectures Paget spoke briefly to the other students in the class and requested their acceptance of her. Dr Blackwell wrote, 'When I entered and bowed I received a round of applause. My seat is always reserved for me and I have no trouble. There are, I think, about sixty students, the most gentlemanly class I have seen.'[21]

Elizabeth Blackwell remained at St Bartholomew's for a year, during which she gained in knowledge and experience. Gratitude for her reception there did not, however, dim her critical faculties. Later she could not help comparing the dull conservatism of English physicians with the lively and innovative style of the French. She herself was also the subject of critical appraisal. Paget kept brief notes on all his students; of her he said, 'The celebrated Dr Elizabeth Blackwell—a sensible, quiet, discreet lady—she gained a fair knowledge (not more) of medicine, practised in New York, then tried to promote female doctordom in England.'[22] In later years the profession would hear more of the promoters of 'female doctordom'.

Family events
The year 1851 was an eventful one for both George and James. In July of that year George was elected Linacre Lecturer in Medicine at St John's College, Cambridge, and in December he gave up the Fellowship of Caius College. The Fellowship had played an important part in his life for nearly twenty years, but one of its conditions was that the holder must be a bachelor. Now, at the age of forty-one, George had become engaged. His marriage to Clara, the youngest daughter of the Revd Thomas Fardell, took place on 11 December, 1851. George had to set about enlarging his consultant practice in order to replace the lost income from the Fellowship, and later to meet his new responsibilities as a family man.

On 20 March, 1851, a second son was born to Lydia and James; they named him Francis. Later in the year James was elected to the Fellowship of the Royal Society, an honour that reflected his growing reputation as a physiologist and pathologist. In July he gave an evening lecture at the Royal College of Surgeons, entitled *The Recent Progress of Anatomy and its Influence on Surgery.* Here he was giving the term 'anatomy' its old comprehensive meaning, which included not only the study of the gross structure of the normal body, but also the elements of the new sciences of histology (the microscopic structure of tissues), pathology, and biochemistry. He said that advances in these new fields would determine progress in surgery:

It would not be difficult to point out a large number of cases in which we may well hope for progress by these means. In regard to such a disease as cancer, for example, we want to know the proportion of cases in which cancer returns after operation, the average time that a patient lives upon whom no operation is performed, the average age, and all other circumstances connected with the disease; and I would venture to say, that whole volumes of statistics as yet recorded upon the matter, nay, that almost every statistical table yet printed is simply and wholly valueless for these purposes, and valueless, chiefly because of the non-use of those means by which alone we can detect what is and what is not a cancer. The microscope must be used, with all other methods of research, before we can approach the knowledge of one of those truths for want of which we are constantly practising in doubt, still casting upon the patient the responsibility we ought to take upon ourselves, still leaving things unsettled which have been unsettled for centuries past.[23]

The value of a scientific training was not to be measured only in terms of factual knowledge; it strengthened the intellect to meet the demands of surgical practice:

We must not forget that the emergencies of surgery are more those of the mind than of the hand. The dextrous hand is indeed a noble gift; he who wears it, wears the best mark of human form, an admirable symbol and instrument of humanity. . . . But much better than the dextrous hand is the instructed mind, clear, strong, resolute, and pliant, experienced in struggles against difficulty—such a mind as can be educated only in the intricacies of some hard science.[24]

Thus it was that the great surgeons of the previous generation—Cline, Astley Cooper, Abernethy, Blizard, and Lynn—had all been pupils of John Hunter, the teacher of anatomy.

Resigns from post as Warden
Towards the end of the year Paget decided, after careful deliberation, to reduce his commitment to the Hospital and to widen the scope of his surgical practice. The success of the College had been achieved at the cost of his physical and emotional reserves. In later life he recalled his responsibilities as Warden, and how fatigue helped him to arrive at a decision that was a landmark in his career:

I took pains to induce some of the best students to be among the first residents, and several complied, including Kirkes and others now gone but not forgotten. But there were, from the first and always, students of all classes; a few idle dissolute fellows whom I had to get rid-of by persuasion or compulsion; others, well-meaning but noisy, time-wasting, troublesome, fond of wine-parties and loud singing, who had to be gently managed, checked, advised, threatened; others, mere triflers, half-willing to work but half ashamed of it, and not knowing how; always wanting guidance and encouragement, seldom improved by it. . . . Seven years' work of this kind was enough for me: I grew older, but the pupils in succession did not; the maintenance of rules became tedious, the anxiety greater; a noisy party, with singing late at night and 'chaffing' of the people in the street, became almost intolerable; and I was glad to have good reason for resigning—the reason, namely, that with children increasing in number it was plain that the income would not be sufficient for their comfort and due training. For this it was essential that I should go into practice where my brass-plate might be in a better place than in Duke Street, Smithfield.[25]

Thus Paget decided to break from his total commitment to the Hospital and to enter into consultant practice. He would retain his appointments as assistant surgeon and lecturer, but would be free to see patients anywhere in London or even further afield. In addition to financial rewards, the change offered a greatly expanded professional experience; he saw it as an essential stage in his development.

But first he had to find a house that would comfortably accommodate his family, and from which he could conduct his practice. Later in the year he heard that a house in Henrietta Street, Cavendish Square, was available for lease on terms he could afford. It had formerly been the home of Sir Thomas Watson, an eminent physician, and was entirely suitable. Thus, in October, 1851, Paget ceased to be Warden of the College and put up his brass plate at 24, Henrietta Street.

Chapter 6

A Liberal Measure of Success

Paget knew that in giving up his post as Warden in order to embark on a career in consulting practice he was exchanging modest security for an uncertain future. For the first year or two he could probably survive on the routine work his friends would send him, but his practice would not be soundly established until strangers, as well as friends, regularly sought his help with their difficult and unusual cases. It could take years to reach this second stage; he could fail and be forced to earn his living as a general practitioner. But he had confidence in his ability to succeed, and even to become one of Britain's leading surgeons.

Having committed himself to a career in consulting practice, he declined a seventh term as the Arris and Gale Professor. Six years previously he had been glad to accept this post at the Royal College of Surgeons as a means of enhancing his reputation. Now circumstances had changed, as he explained to George in a letter:

> The disadvantages [of the Professorship] are that the work necessary to give the lectures well is so great that it leaves me no time for studying such more practical surgery as I find every month more need of knowing. ... But I am very clear that if (D.V.) I work in surgery as I have worked in my other subjects, I can do something in it. There is scarcely any one in England so working—scarcely one who reads a foreign surgical work, or who sets himself to the study with the same resolution and point as one has been obliged to have in studying modern physiology, and such things as I have lectured-on at the College. All advantages of reputation, therefore, seem to be in the surgical direction.[1]

When he reviewed his collected notes for the six courses of Arris and Gale Lectures, it occurred to him that they could form the basis of a textbook of pathology. A year later he had the manuscript ready for publication. Paget's *Lectures on Surgical Pathology,* published by Longmans in 1853, was a popular textbook for many years.

For the first two years his practice fluctuated. Gratifyingly busy periods would be followed by intervals of several weeks during which he saw scarcely a private patient. Meanwhile he had to support his family and contribute his share to the household at Yarmouth. In order to save cab-fares he walked long distances, even in winter, and sometimes arrived at the Hospital for his evening lectures tired and numb with cold. In January, 1853, he suffered another severe attack of pneumonia, from which he allowed himself only the briefest convalescence, for fear of injuring his practice. But as the year progressed there were signs that the worst was over. In 1854 Paget had reason to feel confident that his practice was well established and would continue to grow. The goal he had set himself twenty years before had been reached.

Improved medical training needed

During these early years in practice he did not concern himself with the controversies that stirred the emotions of many of his colleagues. For decades there had been a growing awareness among members of the medical profession of the need for improvement in the system of training and certification of doctors. The Royal Colleges of Physicians and Surgeons, the universities, and the Society of Apothecaries were independent bodies, determining their own methods of training and standards of examination. A layman could not readily distinguish the qualified man from the charlatan, nor could he know which category of doctor was the appropriate one to consult for his complaint. Radical reformers, such as Thomas Wakley, the founder of the *Lancet,* objected to the power of the Royal Colleges; Wakley accused College Fellows of being more concerned with the protection of their status and privileges than with the welfare of the public. The reformers could also point, with justification, to the nepotism that the system of surgical apprenticeship had fostered. The remedy they suggested was the introduction of standardized basic training and certification for all doctors. They also advocated a register listing the names of all qualified medical men, so that members of the public could easily distinguish the trained from the untrained.

Several attempts to introduce legislation incorporating some of these reforms had failed, due in part to the opposition of the Colleges, and in part to lack of agreement between the reformers themselves. Paget believed that the new, non-sectarian, London University should assume responsibility for the training of medical students but, being a loyal Fellow of the Royal College of Surgeons, he preferred to leave the arguments to those who had strong feelings on the subject. Then, in 1854, he became involved in the conflict almost inadvertently, by accepting an appointment as examiner in surgery to the East India Company.

This once immensely wealthy commercial body dominated British trade with the Far East throughout the eighteenth century. In India it had assumed the power and responsibility of a colonial government. But by 1854 the Company had lost its trade monopoly, and the British Government had reduced its administrative power. Nevertheless, senior officers in the Company's service abroad were still regarded as civil servants. The process by which they were selected was subjected to the same degree of public scrutiny as that being applied to Government appointments in general. There was a demand for the setting of minimum standards of education and vocational training, and for formal examinations to replace personal recommendation as the basis of selection of civil servants.

Medical staff selected by examination
To comply with these demands, the Company appointed a panel of four examiners to select medical men for its service abroad. It was announced that Mr Paget would examine in surgery, Dr Parkes in medicine, Mr Busk in anatomy, and Sir Joseph Hooker in general science. Sir Joseph later recalled that it was Paget who took the lead in planning the examinations. There were written and verbal examinations in each subject, and in surgery the candidates were also required to perform a minor and a major operation on a cadaver. Although Membership of one of the three Royal Colleges of Surgery (England, Edinburgh, or Ireland) was a pre-requisite, none of the candidates had ever before been so rigorously examined. Some startling deficiencies in their knowledge were demonstrated. Hooker recalled that several he questioned did not even know the boiling and freezing points of water. Paget was aghast at the ineptitude revealed by the examination in practical surgery.

The examiners failed many of the candidates and advised the East India Company that it should leave several of its vacancies unfilled. They had, in effect, declared the Colleges to be incompetent as examining bodies. The College Councils reacted angrily. The Edinburgh Royal College of Surgeons made a formal complaint to the Government, as a result of which the Company's panel of examiners were called upon to justify their actions. They evidently succeeded, since they were later asked to advise on the selection of medical officers for the Navy and the Army. Paget and Hooker both served on the panel for many years. Hooker later recalled:

> The brunt of the whole fell mainly on Paget: but the result was, that, thanks to him and his method of examining, a great improvement was made in the teaching of Surgery in the Universities and Schools, and a corresponding strictness in the examinations for degrees, etc., followed.[2]

This success could have encouraged Paget to join the campaigners for reform, but he was content to have made his contribution to progress and then to withdraw from the battle. It was in a different context, but probably indicative of his general attitude to reformers, that he wrote: 'No tyranny or injustice can match that of radicals or reformers in a majority. . . . Radicalism is the child of temper more than knowledge or intellect.'[3]

Paget's increasing prosperity

The continuing improvement in Paget's income that began in 1854 was made doubly welcome by the concurrent increase in the size of his family. His third son, Henry Luke, was born in October, 1853; his fourth and last son, Stephen, was born in July, 1856. Despite these extra responsibilities, his financial position towards the end of 1856 was better than it had ever been before. In October James wrote to George:

> At the end of my 'financial year' I find, thank God, an excess of income over expenditure. It is the first time that such an event has ever happened to me. I do not know how to feel thankful enough for this prosperity, and for the hope it brings with it that if God gives me health and strength I may yet work through to the 'owing no man anything' but love. A large share of it will be in my debtor-account with you, long after our money-transactions shall have been justly balanced.[4]

But payment of Samuel Paget's creditors consumed his savings as rapidly as they accumulated. The cheerfulness with which James and George bore this burden for many years is shown in James's letter of 23 September, 1857:

> Thank God I have been able to save enough for this payment without cutting into my October earnings. It is a novel sensation, and a very agreeable one, to find my income surpass my expenses, even though the surplus is thus quickly swept away. The good result of this year is entirely due to increase of practice and I am most thankful to say that the increase is of a kind which I may reasonably hope to go on. Here is my cheque—for the largest sum I ever drew for any purpose of my own—sent with a mixture of regret that it will sweep away all my savings, and of gladness that I have been enabled to save so much. God help us still to obey His own command to owe no man anything but love. For the January payment, I must look chiefly to my October earnings. I will work hard to meet it: and if (D.V.) I succeed, I'll keep a very jolly birthday on the 11th.[5]

Increased recognition for Paget's work

The demands of his practice did not diminish Paget's zeal for increasing his knowledge and carrying out original work in surgery and pathology. An indication of his status in the world of medical science was the recognition accorded him by several international learned societies. In January, 1854, he was elected to the Membership of the Philosophical Society of Philadelphia. Two years later he was similarly honoured by the Société de Biologie de Paris, and by the Société de Chirurgie. In May, 1857, he had the distinction of being invited to deliver the Croonian Lecture to the Royal Society; this is an annual lecture named after a seventeenth-century benefactor of the Society, William Croone.

Death in the Paget household

The title he chose for his Croonian Lecture was *On the Cause of the Rhythmic Motion of the Heart,* but in developing this theme he ranged far beyond the physiology of heart muscle. He considered the accurately regulated sequences of events that cause immature living organisms, both plant and animal, to grow to maturity and then to wither and die. Death, as much as birth, was part of the biological process, he argued. This theme continued to exercise Paget's thoughts for many years, but it had a special relevance at this time. A month before the Croonian Lecture Samuel Paget had died. In the previous year James had observed his father's increasing infirmity and had recognized it as a normal ageing process, unrelated to any form of disease. Writing to George, James spoke of their father's peaceful end:

> This morning brought me the account of our father's death; a solemn, rather than a sad, event; for it would be to wish that we were immortal upon earth, if we were to desire to die otherwise than he has died. He outlived all his griefs: and was, at last, hardly sensible of earthly joy; but it may be a source of great happiness to us that, so long as he could think, he thought happily of us, and that we have been enabled to assist in making the end of his life here serene and free from cares of this world.[6]

Samuel Paget's death ended the family's association with Great Yarmouth. His two daughters moved to Kirstead, in Norfolk, where they lived with their youngest brother, Alfred. Alfred, who was Rector of Kirstead, was a bachelor, so he was pleased to have Patty and Kate to housekeep for him and to assist with the work of the parish.

Notable events that affected Paget both directly and indirectly

Six years after moving to 24, Henrietta Street, Paget found the house no longer large enough to accommodate both his family and his practice. He learned of a larger house, quite close by, that was available for leasing. It was in Harewood Place, between Oxford Street and Hanover Square, and was 'quiet, comfortable, and healthy'. He arranged to move to 1, Harewood Place, early in 1858.

The years in Henrietta Street had been happy ones for the family and professionally rewarding for Paget himself. They were also notable for several historic events that concerned him indirectly. In 1852 the impact of the goldrush to Australia was felt even in St Bartholomew's Hospital. News of the wondrously rich gold deposits being found in Victoria attracted thousands of enterprising young men from Europe and North America. Paget noted that the exodus to the goldfields was depleting London's medical schools. A former St Bartholomew's student who went to Victoria at this time was Anthony Brownless. Brownless was seeking not gold, but a warmer climate that would restore his health. His quest was successful. He became a prominent member of Melbourne's medical and academic circles and, less than three years after arriving in the colony, was appointed to the Council of the recently-founded University of Melbourne. Brownless worked energetically for the establishment of a medical faculty. Remembering James Paget as one of his teachers at St Bartholomew's, he wrote asking his opinion on the curriculum to be instituted. In the event he did not follow Paget's advice, but the correspondence created a link between two medical schools with vastly different backgrounds.

Once more England experiences a cholera epidemic

In the summer of 1854 there was another epidemic of cholera in England, and again St Bartholomew's used two of its wards solely for cholera patients. During the three months of the epidemic more than three hundred cases were admitted to the Hospital; one third of these died of the disease. The high mortality was no reflection on the care given at the Hospital, since most of the deaths occurred in patients who had been brought in from the streets in a moribund condition.

John Snow continued his investigations of the relationship between contaminated water supplies and outbreaks of cholera. He found that in South London two different companies supplying the population's drinking water drew their supplies from different sites in the Thames. The Southwark and Vauxhall Company had its intake works near a sewage effluent; the Lambeth Company had relocated its intake works upstream, where the water was relatively pure. Customers of the Southwark and Vauxhall Company had an incidence of cholera fourteen times greater than that of their neighbours who were supplied by the Lambeth Company. The two companies were, in effect, performing a controlled experiment that demonstrated the significance of the water supply in spreading the disease. Snow observed:

> The pipes of each Company go down all the streets, and into nearly all the courts and alleys. A few houses are supplied by one Company and a few by the other, according to the decision of the owner or occupier at that time when the Water Companies were

in active competition. In many cases a single house has a supply different from that on either side. Each company supplies both rich and poor, both large houses and small: there is no difference either in the condition or occupation of the persons receiving the water of the different Companies. . . . No experiment could have been devised which would more thoroughly test the effect of water supply on the progress of cholera than this, which circumstances placed ready made before the observer.

The experiment, too, was on the grandest scale. No fewer than three hundred thousand people of both sexes, of every age and occupation, and of every rank and station, from gentle-folks down to the very poor, were divided into two groups without their choice, and, in most cases, without their knowledge; one group being supplied with water containing the sewage of London, and, amongst it, whatever might have come from the cholera patients, the other group having water quite free from such impurity.[7]

Another severe outbreak of cholera was localized to an area lying between Regent and Wardour Streets. It began late in August, and by 2 September had caused eighty-nine deaths. Snow found that the incidence of the disease was greater in the vicinity of the Broad Street pump. Further inquiry revealed that, with few exceptions, those who contracted the disease were known to have drunk water from this pump shortly before the onset of symptoms. Snow's investigations led him to conclude that the water of the pump had been contaminated by seepage from an adjacent sewer, so he met with the Board of Guardians of the parish and told them of his findings. The Guardians were sufficiently impressed to order the removal of the pump handle the next day. The epidemic rapidly subsided. Although nearly thirty years were to elapse before Robert Koch discovered the bacterium responsible for cholera, Snow's work had paved the way for public health measures that would prevent further serious outbreaks of the disease. There was a minor outbreak of cholera in London in 1866, but after 1854 there were no more large-scale epidemics.

Florence Nightingale's influence in the Crimea
While London's citizens suffered the cholera epidemic of 1854, British soldiers were fighting and dying on the Crimean Peninsula. In the hopelessly inefficient army hospitals men who had been wounded in battle were dying through neglect and filth. Cholera also contributed to the mortality of the battlefields. In November 1854 Florence Nightingale arrived at Scutari with her party of thirty-eight nurses, and began the transformation that was to make her one of the heroines of history. Paget, who followed her career

and achievements with interest, was one of her staunchest supporters.

After her return to England in 1856 Miss Nightingale threw all her prodigious mental energy into work for the improvement of hospitals, both civil and military. Her health had suffered as the result of exhaustion and an attack of fever while she was in the Crimea, and thereafter she lived the life of a recluse, believing herself to be an invalid. Nevertheless, from her sickroom there flowed an ocean of correspondence—appeals, instructions, and inquiries, directed to people who could help her in her campaigns. Few of these men and women were granted the privilege of meeting her in person. James Paget probably made her acquaintance in 1859, when one of her maids was his patient, and he soon became one of her most trusted advisers. Her books *Notes on Hospitals* and *Notes on Nursing* convinced him that she was well qualified to lead a crusade for improved hospital services. Another of her interests won his approval—her advocacy of statistical records as a basis for the auditing of medical treatment.

In the Crimea Miss Nightingale had been shocked to find that Army hospitals did not even record their deaths with accuracy. Later she found that the London hospitals used a variety of systems for recording diagnoses and results of treatment, so comparisons between institutions were impossible. With the help of Dr William Farr, a statistician in the Registrar-General's Office, she drew up standard forms for hospital use. Then she turned to medical friends for help with introducing the forms into the leading hospitals of London. The response from St Bartholomew's was particularly gratifying, thanks to the influence of James Paget; St Bartholomew's appointed a registrar to deal with the matter and promised a report at the end of the first year.

Paget suggested an extension of the system to include statistics on the results of surgical operations. He was well aware that many doctors failed to review their own cases objectively, so they were not learning from experience. In 1861 he wrote to Miss Nightingale:

> We want a much more exact account and a more particular record of each case. Thus in some returns we have about 40 per cent of the deaths ascribed to 'exhaustion', in others, referring to the same [kind of] operations, about 3 per cent or less; the truth being that in nearly all cases of 'exhaustion' there was some cause of death which more accurate inquiry would have ascertained.[8]

She responded enthusiastically and, after carefully studying the problem, devised a model form. This was discussed at the International Statistical Congress held in Berlin in 1863. The Royal College of Surgeons then appointed a committee to consider the matter. Probably fearing that the statistics could be misused by malevolents, the committee advised against the adoption of Miss Nightingale's system and the matter was dropped. Paget, as a loyal Fellow of the College, did not protest vigorously or publicly but, in characteristic manner, continued to press for more careful self-assessment by his surgical colleagues.

Surgeon Extraordinary to Her Majesty Queen Victoria

Within a few weeks of moving to Harewood Place Paget was appointed Surgeon Extraordinary to Her Majesty Queen Victoria. He had not previously been much in the public eye, so this mark of Royal favour caused a flutter of surprise in London's social circles. It was the first of many honours to be bestowed on him in the decade that followed; he was beginning to enjoy the fruits of success.

In June 1859 he resigned from his appointment as lecturer in physiology at the Hospital, having held the post for sixteen years. The growth of his private practice had made inroads into the time he was able to devote to original work in this subject. Paget was probably ahead of many of his colleagues in perceiving that teaching appointments in physiology should be held by men who were able to make them their major professional commitment; his successor as lecturer in physiology at the Hospital was, in fact, another surgeon, William Savory, who held the post for ten years.

Experimentation on animals

One of the notable features of Paget's physiology lectures had been his use of animal experiments to enable students to see for themselves the phenomena he was describing. Mostly he used small animals, such as frogs, but on one occasion he had a more unusual subject, as one of his pupils (William Turner) later recalled:

> Paget's lectures to his students were much more than verbal expositions. He recognised the importance of appealing to the eye as well as to the ear, and of cultivating and stimulating the power of observation of the class. He exhibited numerous diagrams, and as he expounded his subject he utilised his skill as a draughtsman by drawing freely on the slate. He demonstrated the structure of the tissues and the circulation of the blood under the microscope. The phenomena of circulation of the blood were practically illustrated. His lectures on the heart were timed to correspond with some great turtle-feast in the City of London, and the huge reptile, reposing on the lecture-table, was made the medium of demonstrating the movements of the heart, before being converted into soup to tempt the palate of the citizens. The peristaltic action of the intestines, the presence of chyle, its

absorption by the villi, its transmission by the thoracic duct, the presence of non-striped muscle in the coats of the blood-vessels, the difference in the character of the contraction of striped and non-striped fibres, were all demonstrated in the lecture room. . .[9]

These demonstrations of Paget's were particularly notable because there was very little physiological research being carried out in Britain at that time. Although Hunter had shown that animal experimentation was vital to scientific progress, after his death it was the French and Germans who became the leaders in this field. The use of live animals in experiments was then, and still remains, a controversial subject. Paget's experiments did not provoke a hostile public reaction because they were not performed for public audiences and the animals he used were not cats or dogs, the favourite domestic pets. An episode that occurred in 1824 had shown that opposition could readily be provoked. In that year François Magendie, the French neuro-physiologist, visited England and gave a series of public lectures, which were accompanied by demonstrations on live cats and dogs. There was an outcry at the suffering inflicted on the animals; even a number of scientists thought Magendie strangely callous. Magendie soon returned to France, but the British physiologists, of whom there were not more than half a dozen, were attacked in the press for months after his visit. One who suffered from these attacks was Marshall Hall, the physiologist who encouraged Paget when the latter was struggling to survive in London. The controversy over animal experimentation, or vivisection, did not die out in 1824; it smouldered for forty years and then again captured public attention.

Further academic appointments

In 1860 Paget became a member of the Senate of the University of London. A year later changes at the Hospital led to his promotion there. Resignations from the surgical staff in April and July resulted in his becoming the senior assistant surgeon for three months, and then being promoted to full surgeon. He was forty-seven years old and had been an assistant surgeon for fourteen years. His official status at the Hospital was now equal to that of Thomas Wormald, but in the larger medical world Paget had long since overtaken his old adversary.

In 1863 he was appointed Surgeon-in-Ordinary to His Royal Highness the Prince of Wales. In July, 1865, he was elected to the Council of the Royal College of Surgeons. In the same year he was appointed joint lecturer in surgery at St Bartholomew's Hospital, the other lecturer being Mr Holmes Coote. It was six years since he had last given formal lectures at the Hospital, and he had missed this form of teaching; in a letter to his friend, Sir William Turner, who had recently become Professor of Anatomy at Edinburgh, Paget wrote:

> I am very happy to hear of your large class. I can feel with and for you the immense pleasure of lecturing to full benches of attentive men. Many and great as have been the pleasures that I have derived from my profession, none has been so great as this. And now, after some years' lapse, I have it again: for my surgical class is the largest in London, and larger than it has been at St. B. H. for fully twenty years.[10]

In August, 1868, the British Medical Association held its Annual Meeting in Oxford. Paget presided over the Section of Surgery and, along with six other prominent members of the Association, was awarded the honorary degree of Doctor of Civil Laws of Oxford. In the same week he and James Syme, the noted Edinburgh surgeon, were awarded honorary Doctorates of Medicine by the University of Bonn. Paget's honour was in recognition of his contributions to the science of pathology.

Paget's contribution to the literature
Paget's published articles and lectures during the years 1858–71 give some indication of the reasons why his colleagues regarded him so highly. Some twenty articles on surgery and pathology covered topics ranging from the post-operative care of surgical patients and the treatment of carbuncles, to the clinical features of conditions that we would now call psychosomatic disorders. Three of his papers dealt with diseases of bone, a section of pathology that he found especially interesting. Later generations of doctors who turn to these articles find that they contain much that is still admirable and instructive. When Paget records his observations made at the bedside, at operation, or in the pathology laboratory, and relates these findings to the clinical course of a disease, he is clearly a master of his subject. The years spent in the post-mortem room and the museum had trained him to be an accurate and thoughtful observer, whose knowledge of pathology probably surpassed that of any of his contemporaries in Britain. He was one of the first surgeons to attempt to make an accurate diagnosis by correlating the patient's symptoms with the abnormalities found on physical examination. In his student days it would not have been unusual for a surgeon to think he could diagnose a serious abdominal disorder without so much as turning back the bedclothes to look at the patient's abdomen! Paget helped to change the profession's attitude to diagnosis; this change led to the development of modern clinical surgery.

Some of his writings have not survived the passage of time.

During his lifetime advances in neurophysiology rendered obsolete his ideas on the localization of function in the brain. His philosophical works, such as the paper *The Chronometry of Life,* delivered at the Royal Institute in April, 1859, have little relevance to modern biological science. However, at the time, this paper attracted considerable comment and resulted in an exchange of letters between Paget and Charles Darwin. They became good friends.

One of the papers of this period of Paget's life still appeals to modern readers because much of its commentary applies to human nature in any age. Paget had heard it said that once, when Abernethy entered a lecture theatre, he surveyed the crowd of students waiting to hear him and exclaimed, 'Good God! What will become of you all?' Fifty years later Paget answered Abernethy's rhetorical question, as it applied to a later generation of students. Paget took a close interest in the careers of the men he taught and, as with any natural phenomenon that interested him, he kept notes on most of them. In 1869 he published an article in the *St Bartholomew's Hospital Reports,* entitled, *What Becomes of Medical Students;* in it he reviewed the subsequent careers of 1226 students he had taught during the period 1839–59.

He found that twenty-three had achieved 'distinguished success'. This happy group were described as follows:

> They are classed as having achieved distinguished success who, within fifteen years after entering, gained, and to the end of the time maintained, leading practices in counties or very large towns; or held important public offices; or became medical officers of large hospitals; or teachers in great schools, as the professors of anatomy in Oxford, Cambridge, and Edinburgh, all of whom it was my singular good fortune to have for pupils.[11]

Over half of the whole group had attained a degree of success ranging from 'very limited' to 'considerable'. Near the lower level in this classification was the son of Charles Costerton, Paget's first teacher. He is described as 'silly, idle, dull, but the least vicious of my old master's four sons. He was for a year or two an assistant, but then died of fever in the Hospital.'

Four left the profession in disgrace. One man who lost money speculating in mines was sent to prison for committing forgery. Another who met an even worse end was 'idle, dissolute, extravagant, vulgar and stupid. He scarcely practised and was chiefly engaged on the turf. He was hung for the murder of a friend.'

Of those who left the profession voluntarily, three became actors, four entered the army with commissions and three enlisted as privates. No less than forty-one died as students, seventeen of them with tuberculosis. Eighty-seven died within twelve years of entering practice; many of these deaths were probably due to infectious diseases caught from patients. Two committed suicide.

Perhaps the most heart-warming story is that of 'a well-meaning weak-minded man. He married a prostitute during his pupilage, and went into a very small practice among the poor at Somers Town. But his wife "turned-to", dispensed for him, took in invalids, and kept his house well: and in 1860 he was well afloat.'

Paget concluded his paper with a message that he often gave to students:

> All my recollections would lead me to tell that every student may draw from his daily life a very likely forecast of his life in practice; for it will depend on himself a hundredfold more than on circumstances. The time and the place, the work to be done and its responsibilities, will change; but the man will be the same, except in so far as he may change himself.[12]

Paget was much less reluctant to speak to students about the moral and ethical responsibilities of their profession than modern lecturers seem to be. Reticence about matters of conscience has increased, rather than decreased, in an age which regards any other subject as suitable for frank public discussion. In 1846, and again in 1863, Paget spoke to Hospital students at the beginning of their academic year, warning them of their obligations to those in their care. In 1863 he said:

> Your engagement in this profession binds you, not only by considerations of your own interest, but by the weightiest responsibility to God and man, to do your duty in it with all your might. Keep this constantly in view; daily remind yourselves that you propose to take in hand the lives and the welfares of your fellowmen: daily think quietly of what all this involves; and then you will daily decide that not even your own lives must be much dearer to you than the duties of your profession. . . .

> Experience is of no natural growth in us; it is not commensurate with age. After about thirty, wise men may grow wiser, but unwise men rarely grow wise. Therefore there are many old men with no experience at all. At the right time of life—that is, at your time of life—they did not learn how to learn; and ever since, though working in the field of knowledge—working, it may be, as hard as wiser men—they have been gathering only weeds. Among these are they who, if I may use the sacred allegory, are constantly sowing tares among the wheat of truth. . . .

> You will be tempted to make displays of cleverness; to wish to

seem able to do your whole work, whether in study or in practice, easily and yet well. Why is it that nearly all of us are so much less anxious to be wise than to seem clever? Surely good education should teach us all that nothing good was ever easy. Now, educate yourselves into the dread of being merely clever; for I am sure that anyone who will fairly review the errors of his practice will find that a very large portion of them must be ascribed to his having underrated the difficulty of that which he undertook—to his having tried to be clever when he ought to have been wise. Oh, beware of mere cleverness! . . .

And there is yet another temptation against which I venture to warn you. That which will most harass you in your practice will be the apparent success of dishonesty. You must be prepared for it; for it will not cease in your time, if indeed it ever does. In our department of social life, as in all others, the supply of rogues is duly proportioned to that of fools. For the most part, medical dishonesty is but the complement of non-medical folly. Therefore, until there is a widespread teaching of natural science, there probably will always be much success in quackery. . . .

The burden of my address is work, lifelong work. And so it is, and so it must be; there is no success without it, no happiness without it. A kind of success, indeed, there is without it—the getting of money without honour—and to that there are many ways; but we do not teach them here.[13]

A contented family life

This period of professional achievement was also one of contented family life. In May, 1860, their last child, a daughter, was born to Lydia and James; they named her Mary Maude. James's family thus resembled his father's in that the two girls were the eldest and the youngest of the children, but James and Lydia had the happiness of seeing every one of their babies survive. Their children all outlived them.

The youngest son, Stephen, in later life took on the role of family chronicler, preserving his father's letters and memoirs and adding to them his own recollections of family life. He was middle-aged when he wrote this description of the home of his childhood; in it he mentions his father by name only once, but it is clear that the personality of James Paget was felt in every room of the house.

In the old days, Harewood Place was almost as quiet as the country; there was no thoroughfare, and no noise, only the distant traffic in Oxford Street. The house had its faults; but, for his work, and for home-life, and for hospitality, it was excellent—above all, in summer, when its broad stone staircase and landings kept it cool on the hottest day; the sort of house that is at its best in summer-time, with flowers everywhere, and windows wide open, yet with music undisturbed.

There were only two rooms on the ground-floor, his study and the dining-room, with the width of the hall between them. His study was very plainly furnished, and might have been made more comfortable for his patients: there was no surgical couch, or screen, or looking-glass—nothing to smooth-over or delay the consultation—only straight-backed chairs, and a horsehair sofa of old-fashioned shape. But the room was pleasant to look at; its walls were covered with books and portraits; the places of highest honour were given to John Hunter, Percivall Pott, Abernethy, and Lawrence; and to a portrait of Her Majesty Queen Victoria, that he bought out of the first fee that he received from a Royal patient. Among the things on the mantelpiece was the stethoscope that he bought with his first half-guinea, in the days of his apprenticeship; and, at either end of the mantelpiece, the tall white figures of St Bartholomew and St James, casts from St Sebald's shrine at Nürnberg, that he bought at Oxford in 1844. On the first floor, were the drawing-room and the 'school-room': and his practice, like John Hunter's, often flowed up to this level. In the drawing-room, flowers, and gifts from friends or from patients, were crowded everywhere; he writes to one of his sons, 'Mingling as one may the happiness of looking at the decorations of the rooms, and of remembering the personal stories connected with them, this house is the most charming ever known to me.[14]

The long evenings that Paget shared with his family were recalled by Stephen:

He usually came in about five, for tea and letters. Dinner was a very plain meal, soon over; a Spartan sort of dessert was put-out upstairs; he fetched his books and papers from his study, un-locked his desk, and set to work, at a narrow segment of the table that we all used. Two feet and a half were enough for his desk, his letters, and his glass of wine: and always, year in year out, he sat at the same point of the table's compass, and made the least possible space do for everything. He began work at once: took his wine, and his tea, while he wrote; heard and praised the music, but did not stop writing for it; at 10, read prayers, then wrote till 12, and sent his first batch of letters to the post; then wrote again, or read pathology or surgery, till one or two in the morning. Of all memories of Harewood Place, the most vivid is of him sitting at his own small share of the big round table, at his desk: and we knew the moment when he signed a letter, and the etching sound of his pen changed to a swishing sound as he wrote his name. It is hard to imagine him at a different point of the table, or with his books and papers a foot out of place; and he always declared that he had plenty of room. In the earlier years, if he could not keep awake, he sometimes lay on the sofa and slept; in the later years, he fought sleep at his desk, with good success. He seldom put his work aside for a talk; only, he would sometime take part in such speculative and controversial arguments, about things in general, as are common in families: and if the tide of debate set toward him, even at one o'clock in the morning, he would still be alert, and very careful of his words; and would listen gravely to a lot of rather wild and whirling talk, such as young people think philosophical and final, and would even be one of the disputants; then, later still, he would send the rest of his letters to the post, and his day's work would be done.[15]

The mother's influence on the family was no less than the father's. Lydia Paget led 'a gentle and reverent life' that endeared her to all who knew her. A capable woman who reared healthy children and managed her household without waste or extravagance, she was also generous to those in need. Her tastes in literature were unsophisticated; she was not a brilliant conversationalist, yet famous people enjoyed talking to her because, like her husband, she was an attentive and responsive listener. She sang and played the piano with considerably more skill than most, in an age when ladies were expected to possess such drawing-room accomplishments. Stephen recalled:

Thanks to her, there was always good music to be had for the asking at Harewood Place: especially, at the old-fashioned, informal, hospitable Sunday supper, a very pleasant meal, seldom without friends, and never without music—the one idle irresponsible bit of the week when everybody said whatever he liked. Sometimes, the music and the talk were of the utmost excellence; as when Miss Janotha*, Mr James Knowles†, and Canon Scott Holland, were all there together. And sometimes, but this was a rare event, the talk ousted the music; as when Surgeon Parke came, and told his adventures in Central Africa— one of the younger men in his profession whom my father most admired and honoured.[16]

---

* Miss Janotha was a noted pianist;

† Mr James Knowles was the editor of the journal *Nineteenth Century* .

Lydia Paget was a courageous woman. Stephen tells how on one occasion when she was nursing her husband through an episode of pneumonia, she bent over the bed to give him a drink, and the candle she was holding set fire to the bed curtains. She calmly extinguished the flames with her bare hands, before the patient realized that anything was amiss. Although Lydia seems to have been the perfect wife and mother, Stephen hints that she was not entirely without human weaknesses. On one occasion her sister-in-law, Kate Paget, visited Harewood Place for a small family dinner party in honour of James's birthday. Kate could rarely afford to indulge her taste for fashionable clothes, but on this evening 'she came in a new dress of sky blue and daffodil yellow; it was no mortal dress, it was a heavenly special creation of brilliant and audacious colouring and extravagant beauty and it shabbified the rest of us and sadly offended my Mother'.

In 1861 Alfred Paget died, and Patty and Kate had to find a new home. The little store of treasures saved from the house on the Quay was again packed up, for what was to be their last move. The two sisters settled at Woodridings, near Pinner, in Middlesex, where they shared a cottage with Elise, one of the daughters of their eldest brother, Frederick.

In 1862 George and James paid the last of the bills that had been presented by their father's creditors. James went further and sought out a man who had never pressed for payment; he paid him in full, with accumulated interest. The brothers were at last free of their burden.

A few months previously James had enjoyed his first holiday for seventeen years. He took his wife and daughter Catherine to North Wales for three weeks. He was so delighted to be leaving work behind for a short time that, as they took their seats in the train, he threw his hat in the air like a happy schoolboy.

In 1867 Paget attended the Princess of Wales for a severe and protracted illness. When she recovered and went to Wiesbaden to complete her convalescence, Paget went also, as a member of the Royal household. The famous resort had little to interest him; most of the visitors were rich hypochondriacs, people who had 'nothing to cure but what might be cured by moderate self-denial or borne with moderate patience'. But he enjoyed a scientific conference in Frankfurt, and excursions on the Rhine. This visit to Germany seems to have re-awakened his enthusiasm for foreign travel, dormant since the unhappy sojourn in Paris thirty years before.

In 1868 Paget was able, for the first time, to take a holiday in company with all his family. Thereafter the family went away together each year, sometimes to Wales or Scotland but, whenever circumstances permitted, to the Swiss Alps. Paget believed that a successful holiday was one that left the members of the party refreshed and eager to return to work, rather than sluggish from laziness and self-indulgence. But his somewhat Spartan ideas of enjoyment were entirely acceptable to his family, and soon so many of their friends also joined the party that it resembled a small army setting off from London. Stephen Paget recalled how the holidays were spent:

> He made a rule for his sons, that the holiday should also be a reading-party; except for those holidays that were spent in going

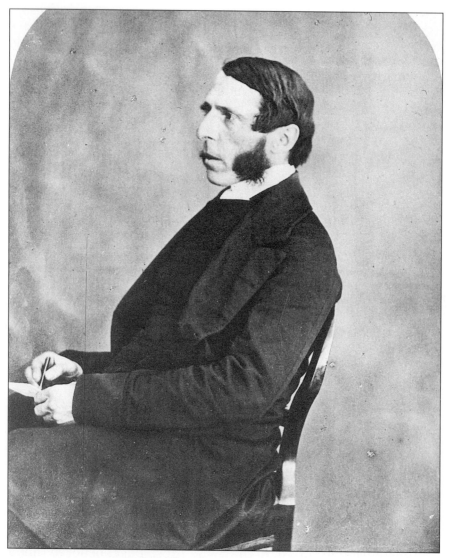

Alfred Paget. (Sir Julian Paget).

from place to place. There was reading all the morning, with one day a week off; and again in the evening, according to age and advancement in learning: law, divinity, logic, Greek and Latin— four or five or six hours a day. He too worked all the morning, usually at a table in the open air, writing letters or lectures. In the afternoon, a long expedition all together; and in the evening, the reading again, and music. But there were times that were holidays indeed, day after day in the open country, walking or driving; and we used to do our twenty miles a day, all together,

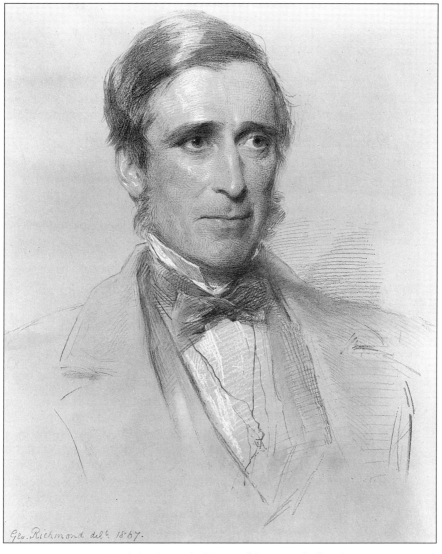

Geo. Richmond delt 1867.

James Paget, 1867. By G Richmond. (National Portrait Gallery).

and mostly on the high-road. At the halt for *mittagessen*, the young men of the party would bathe, if they got a decent chance: and when evening came we would still be walking, even singing part-songs, as we tramped the last miles between us and *abend-sessen*, or shortening the way by some interminable argument. He delighted in these long walks, and in the food taken pic-nic fashion or at wayside inns . . .

He loved all sight-seeing; his enjoyment of a new town was as eager, till he was nearly seventy years old, as his enjoyment of the country. Perhaps he preferred, on the whole, the Simplon Pass, or San Martino, or the road from Landro to Pieve di Cadore: but he got hardly less happiness from pictures, churches, and 'town-scenery' . . .[17]

The pleasures of sight-seeing while on holiday remained with Paget when he returned home. Now that his responsibilities weighed less heavily he had the time to enjoy the sights of London:

He would go to see old City churches; or would walk, on winter evenings, through the shabbiest streets, to see the picturesque effect of lighted fish-stalls and fruit-stalls: he describes, in one of his letters, 'the strange mingling of fog, and brilliant flaring gas, and the colours of fruit and fish and bright metal.' Flowers and fruit, stacked on barrows, or piled-up in cheap shops, gave him a twofold pleasure, by their beauty, and by 'the blessing that such luxuries should be within the reach of the very poorest.'[18]

He enjoyed walking with his children at home in London, as well as when away on holidays:

In the days before he had a carriage, he often walked down to the Hospital: and had at one time the habit of reading as he walked: but he gave this up, after the knocking-down of a small child. On Sundays, carriage or no carriage, he always preferred to walk, and to take some of us with him. We remember his pointing out the barriers set outside Newgate for the public execution of the pirates of the 'Flowery Land'; and his disgust at the sight of a crowd of men and women already, on Sunday morning, waiting to see them hanged. On these visits he used to take us round his wards, but not into all of them; and used to say 'You had better not look at this,' when he came to something terrifying to children; and, if one turned faint, would send him to cool in the Sister's room, or in the Hospital Square. If his visit were in the morning, he attended the service at the Hospital church.[19]

Lister's combat of 'hospitalism'

At the Annual Meeting of the British Medical Association held in Oxford in August, 1868, Paget opened the proceedings of the Section of Surgery with a review of important recent advances. He did not refer to a paper by Joseph Lister that had appeared in the *Lancet* of the previous year. Nevertheless, the ideas expressed in that paper were to transform surgical practice during Paget's lifetime.

The introduction of anaesthesia twenty years previously had removed much of the horror of operations, but surgeons were still reluctant to operate, and there had been no significant widening of the scope of operative surgery. This was because of the frequency of septic complications that caused serious sickness and death in the post-operative period. These complications were much more common in hospital patients than in those who were treated in their own homes, and were therefore referred to collectively as 'hospitalism'. The mortality of hospitalism varied from time to time, and from one institution to another, but was rarely less than 25 per cent, and was often twice that figure. Accidental injuries, such as severe lacerations and compound fractures, were also likely to lead to hospitalism. But it was commonly observed that injuries in which the skin remained intact, such as simple fractures, healed uneventfully.

Any surgical wound was almost certain to suppurate within a day or two. In favourable cases the discharge of pus gradually diminished and the wound eventually healed; the less fortunate passed through a phase of sickness and fever before healing began. Then there were the serious complications. If gangrene set in, the tissues around the wound became discoloured and separated as evil-smelling sloughs. Some patients developed abscesses in sites remote from the wound; this could result in death from a prolonged wasting illness. Sometimes the disease of hospitalism ran an acute course. The patient became cold and shivery, mental confusion rapidly deepened to coma, and death followed within a few hours; the sequence of events suggested that the patient had been poisoned by some substance that had entered the bloodstream.

Every surgeon was familiar with hospitalism, and there were many theories to account for it. Its constant association with skin wounds led to the belief that contact with the atmosphere was the prime cause of suppuration in the deeper tissues. The pus produced in this way acted as an irritant, causing inflammation and gangrene locally, and poisoning the body if it entered the circulation. Some supporters of this theory believed that the oxygen in the air was the agent responsible, but they could not account for the higher incidence of the disease in hospital patients. Others suggested that poisonous vapours were emitted by diseased tissues, and that these vapours were present in much higher concentrations in the atmosphere of hospitals. Attempts to control the disease by improving the ventilation of wards and increasing the spaces between beds had little effect. Some believed that the poisonous vapours had impregnated the walls of the wards, and that old hospitals should be burned down and replaced by new ones.

Important work carried out between 1847 and 1865 by Ignaz Semmelweiss, a Hungarian obstetrician, had gone largely unnoticed. Semmelweiss studied puerperal fever, a disease similar to hospitalism. He concluded that the agent responsible for puerperal fever was carried from diseased to healthy patients on the hands of medical attendants. He succeeded in controlling the disease by insisting that doctors and midwives washed their hands and soaked them in a solution of chlorinated lime whenever they were about to examine a patient.

In Britain the surgeon Joseph Lister sought a means of preventing hospitalism in the wards of the Glasgow Royal Infirmary, where its incidence was very high. Lister was impressed with experiments performed by Pasteur to refute the theory of spontaneous generation. Pasteur found that a piece of wholesome raw meat kept sealed in a glass container did not putrefy until the container was opened and air was admitted. However, if the air entering the container had been filtered so that all particulate matter was removed, the meat remained fresh. It was thus not the gases of the atmosphere that caused putrefaction, but some minute particles that were suspended in it. These minute particles were invisible to the naked eye, although they could be seen with the aid of the microscope. Pasteur went on to show that the particles were living organisms, which could be killed by heat and certain chemicals.

Lister recognized the similarity between the putrefaction of meat and the septic changes occurring in wounds; perhaps hospitalism could be caused by harmful organisms floating in the air and carried into open wounds. If so, it could be combated by cleansing and dressing the wounds with a chemical solution, an 'antiseptic', that killed the micro-organisms. Lister obtained encouraging results when he put his antiseptic method into practice, but for years many of his colleagues were unconvinced, and a few opposed him vehemently.

The antiseptic Lister chose was carbolic acid. If used in too high a concentration it irritated the tissues; hence some surgeons who tried it reported that it was positively harmful. Most of those who claimed to have tested the antiseptic method, and found it useless, had failed to grasp its principles. Leading surgeons, including James Paget, had always stressed the importance of neatness and cleanliness in operating, but they did not appreciate the vital difference between sterility and domestic cleanliness.

In 1867, the year in which Lister's historic paper *On a New*

Method of Treating Compound Fracture, Abscess, etc., appeared in the *Lancet,* the same journal published a series of lectures by James Paget, on *The Various Risks of Operation.* Both authors were concerned with making surgery a safer form of treatment, but their approaches were entirely different. Lister focussed on a single important aspect, that of wound infection and its prevention. He was able to define his problem precisely, and to recommend a solution that was both simple and effective. Paget tackled a problem that defied precise definition, and for which there could be no single solution: the difficulty of estimating the risks of surgery in an individual patient, and balancing those risks against the possible benefits to be obtained. Frail elderly people were, in general, not good subjects for surgery, but sometimes they recovered uneventfully, with their well-being greatly improved by the operation. Obesity, alcoholism, and chronic medical complaints such as syphilis and phthisis (tuberculosis), had to be taken into account when considering surgical intervention. Another important factor was the capacity of the patient to bear fear, pain, and mutilation. It may be necessary to modify the technique of the operation, or to take precautions in some patients that would not be indicated in others. The decision to advise operation required all the scientific knowledge the surgeon could summon to his aid; it also required an understanding of human beings that could not be gleaned from books. Paget appealed to his students not to waste their time as sightseers in the operating theatre, but to devote themselves instead to the careful study of the patients in the wards of the Hospital. Only there could they begin to acquire the wisdom their profession demanded of them.

Paget and Lister were well acquainted and had a high regard for each other. Ten years previously, when both were carrying out experimental work on the pathology of inflammation, they had exchanged letters on some minor differences in the interpretation of their results. In 1869 the *Lancet* published the text of another lecture by Paget, on the treatment of fractures of the leg. In this Paget stated that he had tried Lister's antiseptic method on a case of compound fracture and that it had 'failed altogether to attain its end'. But Paget's article indicated that he had overlooked several of Lister's precepts. Lister felt obliged to write to the *Lancet* pointing this out, but first he wrote privately to Paget, telling him that he regretted the necessity of publicly correcting him, and also offering to demonstrate his method to any St Bartholomew's men who cared to spend some time with him in Glasgow. An assistant surgeon subsequently spent just one day in Lister's wards. The visitor found the brief experience interesting, but was not converted to the antiseptic method.

Serious illness following a post-mortem examination

Two years after these events Paget himself suffered a very serious illness that had many of the features of hospitalism. On Saturday, 4 February, 1871, he performed a post-mortem examination at St Bartholomew's Hospital. The subject was a man on whom he had operated several weeks previously to remove a stone from the bladder. In performing the post-mortem Paget was assisted by two junior members of the Hospital staff—Mr Bloxam, a surgical registrar, and Mr Young, a house surgeon.

Shortly after they began Young accidentally cut his hand; he was sent away to wash the wound thoroughly, and took no further part in the examination. Paget and Bloxam found that their patient's death was due to the presence of pelvic and abdominal abscesses, and to a large collection of pus surrounding one of his lungs. For most of the hour or so that it took to carry out the examination the two doctors had their bare hands immersed in pus.

The following day, Sunday, Paget noticed that he was unusually tired. He felt no better on the Monday, but managed to complete a long day's work. It began with a lecture to the students, in which he demonstrated the findings of Saturday's post-mortem. During the afternoon he was troubled by pain in the left armpit, severe enough to prevent his moving his arm. When he arrived home at 8.30 p.m, after seeing the last of his patients, he knew that he was seriously unwell. Thus began an illness that lasted for more than two months and almost took his life.

Over the next few days he ran a high fever as pain and swelling extended from the left armpit to the left side of his neck and the back of his chest. During the following fortnight he developed several large abscesses in the neck and chest wall. These were drained, with considerable relief of local pain and also of his fever. Then, when he seemed to be recovering, he developed erysipelas, a spreading inflammation of the skin and superficial tissues. This extended widely over his chest, abdomen, and thighs, and once again he ran a high fever. Although he thought at the time that he was quite lucid, his memory of events during the most severe phase of his illness was sketchy. Later, however, he was able to recall the feeling of depression, and that on one occasion he had vehemently attacked his medical advisers. He described the turning point in his illness:

> It was during the erysipelas that my general health suffered most; but my recollection is not clear about anything but the feelings of intolerable restlessness, which nothing but wine or morphia would tranquillise, and of the interest with which for many days I watched the progress of my own case, fancying myself an intelligent observer. At last, after the erysipelas had

been extending for about ten days, and at the end of nearly six weeks from the infection, there came what seemed to me like a crisis. During the night in which my pulse and temperature were at their highest I had a profuse sweating and a profuse flow of urine, such as I never had in my life before; and next day my pulse and temperature had come down to what may be deemed safety-points, and I was conscious of returning health.[20]

His convalescence was interrupted by an episode of the pneumonia to which he seemed to be so susceptible in times of physical stress, but gradually thereafter he returned to normal health.

The *Lancet* published two bulletins on the progress of his illness, and in June it also carried his article entitled *Notes for a Clinical Lecture on Dissection Poisons*. It was based on his own case. In it he postulated that poisons were released by the tissues of the dead man, and that he had absorbed these poisons through the skin of his hands. Although he referred to his disease as an 'infection' he used the term in a general sense, to mean a disease caused by a noxious agent of any kind. That he did not believe that micro-organisms were involved is clear from the following paragraph:

The first thing observed was a few small pustules on the hands, very trivial-looking things, which appeared on the day after the examination, and in the next week or ten days dried without discharging or causing any local trouble. I think they were only local effects of the simply irritant fluids of the body, or of the carbolic acid oil, with which I had uselessly though thoroughly rubbed my hands before beginning my part of the examination. I see no reason for supposing that the material which poisoned me was from any of these pustules.[21]

The modern explanation is that during the post-mortem examination Paget became infected with the bacterium (probably a highly virulent strain of the streptococcus) that had killed his patient. The 'trivial-looking' pustules on his hands marked the sites of entry of the bacteria. Preliminary rubbing of his hands with carbolic acid could not protect him, because the film of antiseptic would have been rapidly washed away by the infected fluids in which his hands were immersed. Indeed, minute abrasions of the skin caused by the rubbing probably facilitated the entry of the bacteria. Lister must have been dismayed when he read Paget's paper, because it showed that one of his most esteemed colleagues was among the many who still had not grasped the principles of his antiseptic procedure.

Paget believed that he was susceptible to the action of the post-mortem 'poisons' because for some years he had not regularly carried out such examinations himself, but had watched while they were done by his assistants. He had thus, he believed, lost his immunity to the poisons. He also thought that being tired and cold at the time had lowered his resistance still further. These factors could be relevant to some types of bacterial infection, but probably not to the one suffered by Paget on this occasion. Immunity to streptococcal infection cannot be acquired by repeated contact with the organism; furthermore, infection with a highly virulent strain is likely to have serious consequences, regardless of such factors as fatigue and cold. It is of interest that Young, who cut his hand at the beginning of the examination and was sent away to attend to the wound, suffered no ill effects; at that stage of the post-mortem examination the large abscesses had probably not been encountered. Bloxam, who assisted at the entire procedure, subsequently became very sick with pleurisy, of a type that could well have been caused by a streptococcal infection. Illnesses like those suffered by Paget and Bloxam had always been a hazard of medical practice. It was not until the early years of the twentieth century that the introduction of rubber gloves improved safety, not only for patients, but also for their doctors.

Chapter 7

Recognition and Rewards

Although Paget seemed to recover completely, the illness he suffered in the first half of 1871 altered the pattern of his life. It reminded him that his physical reserves were declining, and that he could not continue to work as he had when he was twenty years younger. His private surgical practice was probably the largest in England, yet he still attended the Hospital for several hours every day. For the greater part of his life the Hospital had been his spiritual home; he could hardly bear to think of severing his connection with it. But he knew that it was now well served by younger men of talent and character, and that he need not feel that duty bound him to its service. So in May, 1871, Paget resigned from the staff of St Bartholomew's Hospital.

The Board of Governors received his resignation with great regret. They appointed him a consultant, or permanent adviser, to the Hospital, and on 4 July the Prince of Wales, as President of the Board, formally thanked him for his outstanding service. His colleagues commissioned the artist John Millais to paint his portrait. One of his last house surgeons, Adam Young, later wrote:

> The Millais portrait is a telling likeness of what he was in those days; but I think it shows signs of the dreadful illness he had just passed through; and there is a sadness in the expression which I don't recollect was usual with him; for he was about to give up his work at the Hospital, to which he was so passionately devoted, and all who were intimately acquainted with him know what a grief and trouble this was to him. I do not recollect his ever allowing his private work to interfere with his keeping his appointments at the Hospital: I know on many occasions he had infinite trouble in doing so. We always looked forward to his visits on Sundays; we had him all to ourselves then, and I well remember with what delight we used to listen to him as he talked to us, generally standing in front of the Ward fire.
>
> He expected us to take the greatest pains with all the details of our work, and he held the House-surgeon personally responsible for the state of the Wards and the condition of the patients. He used to preach to us, on all and every occasion the importance of absolute, painstaking, cleanliness in the treatment of surgical

injuries; and, of as much importance, the gentle handling of wounds. Another point he was most particular about, was the comfortable placing of injured limbs; and he encouraged in every way the invention and contriving of appliances to this end. I believe plaster of Paris was first used in his wards: at least I remember when I was a dresser, on one occasion when the Prince and Princess of Wales were going round the wards with him, he

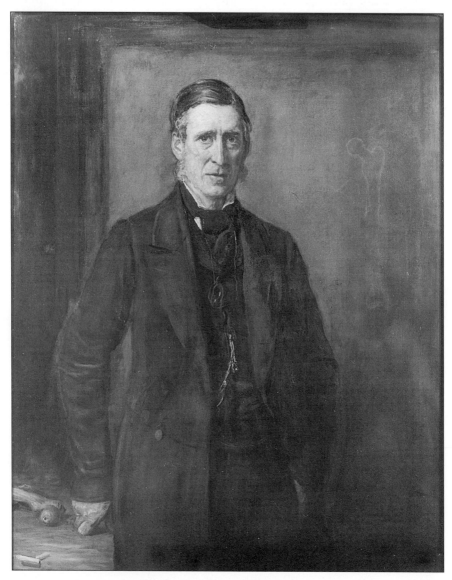

Sir James Paget, 1871. By JE Millais. (St Bartholomew's Hospital).

drew attention to a plaster of Paris bandage I had made, as quite a new thing.[1]

The Paget tradition had been established at St Bartholomew's Hospital; it is still felt by students entering the school more than a century later.

Sir James Paget

A few weeks later the Queen conferred on him a baronetcy, an honour he accepted with pride and pleasure. On his coat of arms he had the old family motto that he and his brothers had made rueful jokes about in their childhood: *Labor ipse voluptas* (Work itself is pleasure). Paget wondered if his colleagues would regard the baronetcy as a sign that he was retiring from practice. He need have had no fears on this score; now that he had more time to devote to it his practice grew even larger.

It amused him to discover that he had become 'fashionable'. On one occasion when the pressure of work delayed his departure for a holiday with the family, he wrote to his wife, 'Tomorrow I have to see a Baron, a Viscount, a Countess, and a Marquis! Cock-a-doodle-Doo'. He was equally amused by the popular saying that those who sought the very best in surgical care went to Paget for the diagnosis, and to Fergusson to have the offending part cut out.

Business-like consultations

The success of physicians in private practice depended to a considerable extent on their 'bedside manner'. The two leading physicians of the seventies, Sir William Jenner and Sir William Gull, each had his loyal adherents, some preferring the brusqueness of Jenner, others the reassuring manner of Gull. One lady was heard to say that she favoured Gull because, instead of prescribing unpleasant medicine, he advised her to take strawberries and cream![2]

Surgeons had a different relationship with their patients. They usually dealt with urgent problems; when these had been overcome their patients were either discharged or returned to the care of physicians. Surgeons were thus not obliged to indulge the foibles of their clientele. Paget's manner with his patients was courteous but business-like. Stephen Paget describes his father's consulting room at Harewood Place as being austerely furnished, with nothing added specifically to give his patients a sense of luxury. Time was precious to James Paget; irrelevant conversation in the consulting room was discouraged:

In the years of heaviest practice, when he often had twenty or more people to see him in the morning, he was sometimes almost exhausted at the end of the time: it was work of the utmost responsibility, and must not be trifled with; one of his children once dared to 'dress up as a patient,' and was shown-in to him, but got no encouragement to do it again. His manner toward new patients was rather formal: it was an ordeal, for some of them, to consult him. He used to stand while he spoke to his patients; and was sparing of his words, but was careful to write or talk fully and precisely to the medical man who had advised or brought the patient to consult him. With those patients who talked much, he was silent: he said it was the quickest way in the end: and he was fond of trying in how few words he could write or say a thing. Once, he was challenged to a sort of contest in brevity, and accepted the challenge; his adversary was a Yorkshireman, who came into his consulting-room, and merely thrust out his lip, saying 'What's that?' 'That's cancer,' he answered. 'And what's to be done with it?' 'Cut it out.' 'What's your fee?' 'Two guineas.' 'You must make a deal of money at that rate.' And there the consultation ended.[3]

If his patients, through weakness or stupidity failed to follow his instructions, he reprimanded them severely. Some actually feared him. Yet those who were seriously ill or troubled knew how compassionate he could be. One of his last assistants at the Hospital recalled:

His tenderness to the patients was a lesson to us all; when he had to say an unpleasant thing to a patient, his gentle sympathetic manner took out much of the sting and sorrow. If he had a poor patient leaving the Hospital, who was in want, I have seen Paget go back, after we were supposed to have gone away, and give him a handful of silver, never troubling to see how much there was.[4]

When it became known that Paget sometimes treated private patients free of charge a few younger surgeons objected. In the seventies the medical profession was so overcrowded that there were doctors who were reduced to selling soap and perfume. Successful men who did not always charge their patients were accused of disloyalty to their struggling colleagues. Paget defended his right to charge or not, as he saw fit, but also supported the cause of doctors who were being exploited by friendly societies and other organisations that sought their services for a pittance. He acquired such a reputation for honesty and discretion in his dealings with colleagues that he was often asked to adjudicate in disputes between members of the profession.

Continued family success
Three of James Paget's four sons chose careers other than medicine.

In 1872 the eldest, John, was completing his Arts and Law degree at Cambridge; he was then to proceed to the Inner Temple to become a barrister. Francis and Henry were both at Oxford studying for Arts degrees before entering the Church. Stephen, who was then still at Shrewsbury School, later became a surgeon and noted author.

George Paget had gained a number of distinctions since giving up his Fellowship of Caius College. Although he was no longer directly involved in College affairs he was increasingly active in the cause of science and medicine at the University. In 1856 he was elected to the Council of the Senate. In 1863 he was appointed the University's representative on the General Medical Council, and six years later he was elected President of the Council. At the conclusion of his five-year term he was unanimously elected for a second term, but he resigned shortly afterwards because of ill-health and pressure of work. He was President of the British Medical Association in 1864. In 1872 he was appointed Regius Professor of Physic in the University of Cambridge, an honour that reflected the high regard the profession had for this able yet unassuming man. His marriage and family life were happy. Clara bore him ten children, of whom seven survived to adult life.

Contributions to the literature continue
For James Paget the decade that followed his retirement from the Hospital was one of undiminished original work. He wrote numerous articles on a wide range of topics including cancer, syphilis, typhoid, acute surgical conditions, and psychological disorders that mimic physical disease. In 1875 he published a collection of his papers under the title *Clinical Lectures and Essays*. Two years later this work was translated into French, and in 1879 a second English edition appeared. Two of the articles he wrote during this period are the ones for which he is now best known.

Paget's disease of the nipple
In 1874 the St Bartholomew's Hospital Reports contained his article entitled *On Disease of the Mammary Areola Preceding Cancer of the Mammary Gland*[5]. In this he reported a series of fifteen cases of chronic ulceration of the nipple occurring in women aged between forty and sixty. The ulcers resembled those that were seen in other areas of the body in several chronic benign skin diseases. But in every one of the cases in this series cancer had appeared in the affected breast within two years. He suggested that the ulcer caused chronic irritation of the breast tissue, and that this in turn led to the development of cancer. It is now known that Paget's disease of the nipple is a manifestation of a cancerous growth already present in the breast. Tumour tissue grows in

microscopic fronds along the lining of the ducts of the breast until it reaches the nipple. Then it invades the skin and causes ulceration. The tumour deep in the breast may be difficult or impossible to detect by physical examination at the stage when the ulcer first appears.

Osteitis deformans—Paget's disease of bone

Two years later, in November, 1876, Paget published in the *Medico-Chirurgical Transactions* a paper with the title *On a Form of Chronic Inflammation of Bones (Osteitis Deformans)*[6]. In this he described five cases of a previously unrecognized disease. His illustrative case was that of a man whom he had first seen in 1854, and whose condition he had observed for twenty years. The patient was forty-six years old when he first consulted Paget, with the complaint of aches and pains in the lower limbs; his general health was otherwise good. Paget observed that the patient's left shin bone was enlarged and deformed and the left thigh bone, although more difficult to feel, seemed to be similarly affected. Careful examination did not reveal any other abnormality. The condition was not one Paget had seen before and he was not able to make a diagnosis.

He described how, in the years that followed, the bones of the man's right leg also enlarged and the legs became bowed, so that it was impossible for him to bring his knees together. The skull enlarged progressively, causing him to buy larger and larger hats as the years passed. He became stooped, so that his head sank on to his chest, and his height decreased by four inches. Despite these changes in his bones his general health remained quite good for his age. Then, twenty years after he had first consulted Paget, the patient noticed a rapidly enlarging bony mass in his left forearm. A bone cancer had developed, and it was this that caused his death two months later.

At the post-mortem examination the presence of a malignant bone tumour in the left forearm was confirmed. Deposits of tumour tissue were found in the chest and skull. The bones that had been observed during life to be abnormal were the only ones found to be affected by the deforming disease. The bones of the right thigh, the left shin, and the upper part of the skull were removed for microscopic examination. This was performed by Mr Henry Butlin. Butlin, who was then a surgical registrar at St Bartholomew's Hospital, had been Paget's house surgeon. It seems likely that it was he who performed the post-mortem examination, and that it was carried out at the Hospital in Paget's presence.

Microscopic examination of the diseased bones revealed an extraordinary aberration of the process of remodelling that normally continues throughout life. Normal bone has an orderly architectural pattern in which at some sites bony substance is being

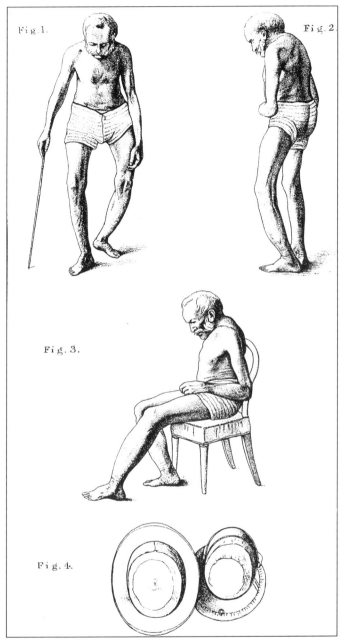

*Illustrations Accompanying Paget's First Article on Osteitis
Deformans. Figs 1–3 are from photographs of the patient
(Case 1) taken six months before his death. Fig 4 is from
photographs of the same patient's cap worn in 1844, and hat
worn in 1876.*

absorbed, and at others new bone is being laid down. By this means the skeleton is constantly being renewed; its strength is also being adjusted to meet the changes in mechanical stress that accompany such phenomena as ageing and prolonged inactivity during sickness. In Paget's patient the remodelling process in the abnormal bones had run riot. Excessive absorption of bone had been followed by disorderly and continued production of new bone in excessive amounts. Thus the bones had become abnormally large. The improperly formed new bone was structurally weak; it bent under the weight of the body, causing the legs to become bowed. Paget thought the process was probably inflammatory in nature, so he called it *osteitis deformans,* or 'deforming inflammation of bones'. The disease is no longer thought to be an inflammation, but modern science has not been able to discover a satisfactory explanation for it.

Forty years after Paget first described his disease of bone, the advent of X-ray techniques enabled the whole skeleton to be observed in the living patient. It was discovered that Paget's disease of bone is not, as he had thought, a rare condition; many older people have one or several bones affected with it and are quite free of symptoms. Paget recorded that in three of his five cases cancer developed in one of the abnormal bones. It was only in this regard that his small series was not a representative one; cancer has proved to be an uncommon complication of Paget's disease of bone.

The microscopic changes seen in Paget's disease of bone and of the nipple

Paget's paper includes an excellent description of the microscopic appearance of the abnormal bones, but this section of the paper was contributed by Butlin, who received due acknowledgement. There is no report of the microscopic findings in his article on ulceration of the nipple although, having operated on two of these patients, he would have had suitable tissue available. These are striking omissions on Paget's part, since he had been one of the first to become skilled in the use of the microscope and was convinced of its importance to the study of pathology. In 1851, when speaking on this subject at a meeting of the Royal College of Surgeons, he had said, 'The microscope must be used, with all other methods of research, before we can approach the knowledge of one of those truths for want of which we are constantly practising in doubt.'[7] Yet it seems that twenty years later he had ceased to use it himself.

There were probably two reasons for this. Firstly, after his resignation from the Hospital he would not have had ready access to the laboratory facilities necessary for the preparation of microscope slides. Secondly, and more importantly, pathology was advancing so rapidly that it was no longer possible to be expert in this field and also actively engaged in clinical practice. Indeed, the time was rapidly approaching when pathologists would be specialists in their own right, providing the skilled diagnostic service their clinical colleagues needed. In his later years Paget's contributions to medical knowledge were the fruits of his experience in the consulting room and the operating theatre, rather than the laboratory.

It is of interest that two years after Paget's disease of the nipple was first described, Henry Butlin published a paper in which he reported the microscopic findings in two cases. He was particularly interested in the relationship between the ulceration and cancer, but could find none:

> . . . There was not any structure in the sections which I could convince myself had reached the condition of actual carcinoma. . . . There being no cancer present in these breasts it is impossible to say that cancer would have formed in either.[8]

It seems highly probable that Butlin showed the slides to Paget, and that they agreed on this interpretation. We now know that in its early stages this disease appears deceptively benign, although modern pathologists readily recognize its malignant nature. Nevertheless, these two papers by Paget are deservedly famous. His ability to delineate the significant features of an obscure disease and to recognize their appearance in another patient, sometimes many years later, is a rare gift. Paget was also able to record his observations so precisely that his original descriptions of these two conditions could not be bettered. Thus we still speak of 'Paget's disease of the nipple' and 'Paget's disease of bone' in an age when most eponyms have been replaced by descriptive scientific terms.

Numerous influential friends

After living austerely for so long Paget found that one of the joys of his later years was the widening of his circle of friends. In his youth his few associates were, of necessity, mainly Hospital men and medical editors. In middle age, as his horizons widened, he made many new friends. Some he met in the conduct of his practice, others while serving on professional and charitable committees. He joined several London clubs; although he could not spare the time to visit them frequently, they introduced him to men who were prominent in literary and political circles. Other friendships grew from an initial meeting to discuss one of his lectures or published articles. This was how he came to know Charles Darwin. Paget's 1859 lecture, *The Chronometry of Life,* led to an exchange of letters and an association that continued until Darwin's death in 1882. Stephen Paget said that his father always regarded himself as

Darwin's disciple, a gatherer of information that the great scientist could use in his work. But Paget's letters suggest that the friendship was evenly based and mutually enjoyable. In a letter written in July, 1875, Paget discusses fairy rings—the strange circles of discolouration that sometimes appear overnight in grass lawns. They are now known to be due to the growth of a fungus in the soil, but Paget was intrigued by their resemblance to some diseases of humans:

> My dear Darwin—Pardon my writing on a railway, and let me thank you for your book on Insectivorous Plants: the more at this time because, while reading it, I have been thoroughly enjoying myself in what might have been a very dull long journey. But neither my reading nor my thanks are yet ended. I am charmed with your suggestion that fairy-rings illustrate the insusceptibility of soils—whether bloods, tissues, or earths—that have been infected. I have sometimes vaguely thought so, but you make me nearly sure. I have been told that fairy-rings sometimes appear very quickly—large and complete rings appearing where no small ones were before. I do not know if this ever happens, and I must admit that my informant ascribed the occurrence to electricity: but he said he had observed it on his own lawn. If such rings are ever complete from the first, I have thought there might be mutual illustrations between them and some forms of annular diseases which one sees in the skin. Some forms of Herpes are from the first annular: still more often some forms of Psoriasis, and of ulcers; and when these begin in rings or parts of rings, they usually extend only outwards, and if they meet they coalesce but do not cross. I will try to get some one to work this out. And, I will not forget your wish for cases of re-growths of amputated members. —Always sincerely yours, James Paget.[9]

Huxley and Pasteur, too, were among Paget's scientist friends. There were also many who were neither scientists nor doctors. His long and close association with William Gladstone began in 1846, when both men were working for the establishment of the House of Charity, a shelter for the poor and homeless in Soho. They had taken turns in sleeping at the House until a resident warden could be appointed. Their friendship endured for fifty years.

A very different personality was Cardinal Newman, whose simplicity and gentleness appealed to Paget. He said of Newman, 'I should think him the most persuasive man I have known. If I had not had an education in science, and learnt the exceeding danger of deductions, and the right and need of doubting all that has not clear evidence of fact or revelation, I should think it dangerous to see him.'

George Eliot and other literary friends

Among his friends from the literary world were George Eliot, Tennyson and Browning. George Eliot, whose real name was Marian Evans, probably met Paget in 1869. She was then fifty years old, and living in a relationship that she regarded as marriage, with the scholar George Lewes. Paget's professional assistance was sought when Thornton, Lewes's son by his wife Agnes, became severely ill. The young man was suffering from spinal tuberculosis, which caused his death six months later. Marian and George Lewes thought that Paget had not at first realized the severity of Thornton's disease or arrived at the correct diagnosis. It seems more likely that he was reluctant to tell them bluntly that the young man's plight was hopeless. Although the tubercle bacillus had not then been discovered, the various manifestations of the disease were so well known that a skilled diagnostician like Paget could hardly have been mystified by a typical case.

Marian and George Lewes became friends of the Pagets. James rarely read fiction, but he made an exception of George Eliot's novels. She always sent him a copy of her latest work and the arrival of one of these was one of the very few excuses he would allow himself for postponing an evening's work. When her writing touched on medical matters she usually sought Paget's advice, so that she could be sure of avoiding technical errors. She omitted to do this when she was writing a section of *Middlemarch,* and was mortified to have a reader point out a supposed mistake; she had described Lydgate as having 'bright, dilated eyes' after he had taken opium, when in fact opium causes the pupils to become constricted. She appealed to Paget for advice. He replied that she had not really been in error. Excitement could cause the eyelids to be retracted, giving a staring expression as she had implied, even though the pupils were constricted by opium. However, in later editions of the novel she changed the wording so that there could be no misunderstanding.

Late in 1878 Paget was consulted by George Lewes, who was suffering severe pelvic pain. The symptoms were found to be due to advanced disease (probably bowel cancer) that would soon have a fatal outcome. Paget did his best to comfort and support the family and was with them when Lewes died a few weeks later.

Marian was beside herself with grief. In her bereavement she was helped by her many friends, but especially by John Cross, a man twenty years her junior. Eighteen months after George Lewes's death Cross asked Marian to marry him. Her feeling for him had changed from friendship to love, but she did not trust her own judgement in making such an important decision. In her anxiety she turned to Paget for advice. He gave her the reassurance she needed, and four weeks later Marian Evans and John Cross were married. The marriage gave both of them a few months of happiness before Marian died, on 22 December 1880. Lydia Paget wrote of her:

> The more one thinks of her, and her deep affection for your father, the more one feels how she stood alone, amid the many friends he has won. I never can think of her without a strange feeling of jealousy over her, a kind of true regard and admiration I can't describe. She was so gentle, so generous, so affectionate, so charitable in her spirit towards others.[10]

Paget revered Tennyson, although he admitted that he had had 'to read and write too much of plain descriptions, too many catalogues', to be able to appreciate Tennyson's poetry. Browning and Paget had many mutual friends; when they gathered at Harewood Place there was sure to be good conservation. A friend wrote this description for Stephen Paget:

> I can now see your father, with Browning on one side, and

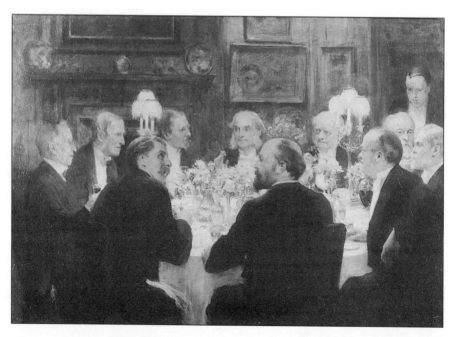

An Octave for Mr Ernest Hart. By SJ Solomon, 1894 . (Wellcome Institute).

Octaves were dinner-parties held by Sir Henry Thompson Bt, at his house at 35 Wimpole Street, at which eight courses, accompanied by eight wines, were served at eight o'clock to eight guests in addition to the host and guest of honour. Clockwise from the centre background (right of mantelpiece):

Romanes on the other, telling stories about the appearance of the stigmata—(there had been a girl in Belgium who had attracted much attention by her claim to this manifestation)—then, about blushing—then, about electrical fishes—and, last, a story of Browning's, of a girl in their lodgings somewhere in Italy, who they found regularly stole their tea, which they bore with, but rebelled when they found that she likewise stole their candles, yet were mollified when they found out that she stole their candles in order to burn them before a little shrine in expiation of her sin of stealing their tea! These are some of the settings in which your father's keen, firm face and quick eye still look at me.[11]

Paget's early educational deficiencies were no bar to his social life

Paget thought that his education at Mr Bowles's school had left him unprepared for social life, but his friends did not share this opinion. The seriousness that characterized his attitude to work disappeared when he was enjoying a good dinner in the company of

---

Ernest Abraham Hart (1835–1898) MRCS. Surgeon, editor of the British Medical Journal *1870–1898, promoter of sanitary improvements. Guest of honour at the* Octave.

Sir Thomas Spencer Wells (1818–1897), 1st baronet (1883), PRCS. Gynaecological surgeon.

Sir Joseph Fayrer (1824–1907), 1st baronet (1896), FRCP, FRS, FRCS. Surgeon-general, Indian Medical Service, authority on snake venom.

Newman, butler to Sir Henry Thompson (in background).

Sir Thomas Lauder Brunton (1844–1916), 1st baronet (1909), FRCP, FRS. Physician, teacher of pharmacology and therapeutics.

Sir William Henry Broadbent (1835–1907), 1st baronet (1893), FRCP, FRS. Physician.

Sir George Anderson Critchett (1845–1925), 1st baronet (1908), FRCS (Edin). Ophthalmic surgeon.

Sir Victor Alexander Haden Horsley (1857–1916), knight bachelor (1902), FRS, FRCS. Surgeon, pathologist, and physiologist.

Sir Richart Quain (1816–1898), 1st baronet (1891), FRCP, FRS. Physician.

Sir James Paget (1814–1899), 1st baronet (1871), FRS, PRCS. Surgeon and pathologist.

Sir Henry Thompson (1820–1904), 1st baronet (1899), FRCS. Urological surgeon, supporter of astronomy and of cremation of the dead, patron and practitioner of arts and letters. Creator and host of the Octaves.

friends; he could match witticisms with the brightest of them. He was frequently included in Sir Henry Thompson's famous Octaves. Thompson, who was a surgeon, was also a dietitian and a gourmet, with a preference for French and Italian cuisine. He gave dinner parties to which he usually invited eight guests, and at which eight courses were served, hence the name 'Octave'. They were noted as much for the brilliance of the conversation as for the excellence of the food and wines.

President of the Royal College of Surgeons of England
The year 1875 brought Paget another professional honour, with its associated burden of responsibility, when he was elected President of the Royal College of Surgeons. He had become a Member of the College in 1836, a Fellow in 1843, and had been on the Council since 1865; for the two years before his presidency he had been Vice-President. He was thus well acquainted with College affairs and with the men who made up the Council. Nevertheless he did not have an easy task. Negotiations were in progress with a view to establishing a Conjoint Board representing the Royal Colleges of Physicians and Surgeons. The proposed Board would conduct examinations and issue combined diplomas in medicine and surgery, thus providing a single basic qualification for medical practitioners.

Paget supported the proposal, but some Fellows of both Colleges were opposed to it. There were also difficulties with the Society of Apothecaries. Paget could not hope to solve these problems during his year in office; indeed, another ten years were to pass before the Conjoint Board became a reality. In 1876 Paget was succeeded as President of the Royal College of Surgeons by Mr Prescott Hewitt, but he exchanged that role for a similar one by becoming the *Medico-Chirurgical Society's President for that year.

Antivivisection
After 1870 Paget found himself increasingly involved in the antivivisection controversy. In that year the Royal College of Surgeons began reforming its examination procedures along the lines advocated by Paget during his service for the East India Company; surgical candidates would henceforth be required to have a much more comprehensive knowledge of physiology. The medical schools were obliged to appoint appropriately qualified lecturers, and to provide them with improved facilities for animal experimentation. In the same year two universities made their first senior academic appointments in physiology. At the University College, London, Burdon-Sanderson was made Professor of Practical Physiology and

---

* Now the Royal Society of Medicine

Histology, with EA Schafer as his Assistant Professor. Trinity College, Cambridge, appointed Michael Foster its first Praelector of Physiology. These eminent men attracted to their institutions scholars who were eager to participate in research. After lying dormant for nearly half a century, British physiology had suddenly burst into activity.

The antivivisectionists did not fail to observe that these developments were causing a dramatic increase in the number of animal experiments performed in England. The Royal Society for the Prevention of Cruelty to Animals, which had been founded in 1824 to deal with the treatment of animals in industry and sport, was not prepared to take a stand against the scientists. The antivivisectionists therefore decided to form their own organisation. The spirit behind the Victoria Street Society, as it came to be called, was a middle-aged woman journalist, Frances Power Cobbe. Miss Cobbe, who had been active in the feminist movement, concentrated her very considerable energy and organizing talent on the antivivisection campaign. She recruited as patrons for her Society the Earl of Shaftesbury, the Archbishop of York, Cardinal Manning, Lord Chief Justice Coleridge, and the poets Tennyson and Browning. In 1875 Shaftesbury became the Society's first President. The Queen herself supported their aims and repeatedly urged her Prime Minister, Benjamin Disraeli, to take action on the matter.

The defenders of animal experimentation were not nearly as well organized as their opponents. Those who performed experiments were a relatively small group; most doctors were not personally affected by the controversy. Some joined the defence only because they resented any attack on the profession. A few members of the medical profession actually supported the antivivisectionists; Sir William Fergusson was one of these. (Some of his critics said that his stance merely reflected the inadequacy of his own training in physiology.)

Sometimes the scientists' actions were detrimental to their own cause. A work entitled *A Handbook for the Physiological Laboratory,* which was published in 1873, put a powerful weapon into the hands of the antivivisectionists. The book was edited by Burdon-Sanderson. Its main contributors were the well-known scientists Michael Foster of Cambridge; T Lauder Brunton, pharmacologist of St Bartholomew's Hospital; and Emanuel Klein, histologist and microbiologist of the Brown Institute. In the introduction Burdon-Sanderson stated that the book was intended for 'beginners'. It gave detailed instructions for the performance of dozens of the classic experiments in physiology, and contained over one hundred illustrations of the animal 'preparations'. There was no mention of the use of anaesthesia, nothing to indicate that the authors felt the slightest concern for the suffering of the animals. The book seemed to provide clear evidence that not only were the scientists themselves utterly callous, but that they were also encouraging untrained students to engage in the wanton destruction of animals.

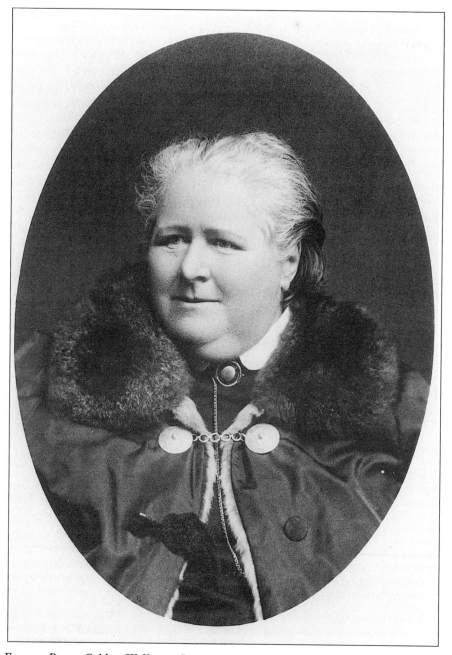

Frances Power Cobbe. (Wellcome Institute).

The Handbook was widely quoted in the lay press and won support for the antivivisectionists.

Queen Victoria takes a view on vivisection
By July, 1875, the controversy had become sufficiently heated to warrant a Royal Commission. The Commission's task was to determine the extent to which animals were being used in laboratories, the importance of these experiments to scientific progress, and whether legislation should be introduced to control the activities of scientists.

The Queen was delighted that at last something was being done. She instructed her private secretary to write to Lister, requesting his assistance:

BALMORAL.
June 15, 1875.

DEAR SIR,
You are no doubt aware that a Royal Commission is about to inquire into the subject of Vivisection, but some time must elapse before any legislation is attempted.

In the mean while it is to be feared that the unnecessary and horrible cruelties which have been perpetrated will continue to be inflicted on the lower animals.

The Queen has been dreadfully shocked at the details of some of these practices, and is most anxious to put a stop to them.

But she feels that no amount of legislation will effect this object so completely as an expression of opinion on the part of some of the leading men of science who have been accused, she is sure unjustly, of encouraging students to experiment on dumb creatures (many of them man's faithful friends and to whom we owe so much of our comfort and pleasure) as a part of the regular educational course.

The Queen therefore appeals to you to make some public declaration in condemnation of these horrible practices, and she feels convinced that you will be supported by many other eminent Physiologists in thus vindicating the Medical Profession and relieving it from the accusation of sanctioning such proceedings.

Yours faithfully,
HENRY F. PONSONBY.[12]

Lister regretfully declined the request. In his lengthy reply he referred to many instances of cruelty to animals that passed unchallenged, although the pain was inflicted for unworthy or trivial motives:

> All oxen and the great majority of our male domestic animals such as sheep, pigs, and horses, have been subjected to an operation involving exquisite agony in its execution, and often severe pain from subsequent inflammation in the wound, the object being to make them more easily fattened for slaughter, their flesh more fitted for human food, or in the case of the horse to render them more patient and docile servants. Compared with practices like these, that which has received the odious appellation of vivisection is justified by far nobler and higher objects; not the ministering to the luxury or comfort of a generation, but devising means which will be available throughout all time for procuring the health of mankind, the greatest of earthly blessings, and prolonging of human life.[13]

Lister believed that the pain felt by some animals was probably less than the onlooker might think, and he was sure that scientists took care to reduce their suffering to a minimum. He concluded:

> I am therefore clearly of opinion that legislation on this subject is wholly uncalled for; while any attempts of that kind might prove very injurious by checking inquiries calculated to promote the best interests of Her Majesty's subjects.

The role of animals in future medical advances
The Victoria Street Society and their supporters had a well-prepared case to put before the Commission. The scientists had to marshall their forces in haste. Men like Paget, Lister, and Gull, who were well known and respected, were to lead the defence. They were conscious of their onerous responsibility. Internal medicine and surgery both stood at the threshold of important advances. Physicians had learned the value of physical signs and had become skilled in the use of the stethoscope. Surgeons had anaesthesia to simplify their task and were optimistic that wound infection would soon cease to be a problem. But neither group could begin to realize the full potential of these innovations without a much more comprehensive knowledge of physiology, pathology, and microbiology. This knowledge could be gained only by direct observation and experimentation. Deductive reasoning, once the only method of research, was no longer acceptable; the testing of every theory, the solving of every problem, called for carefully designed experiments on living animals. If the use of animals were to be severely restricted British medical science would be paralysed.

Paget was not a sentimental animal-lover. He made sure that his coach horses were well treated, but he had no fondness for domestic pets. Although he did not share the feelings of the antivivisectionists, he could understand their concern. He also knew how easily the public could be stirred by accounts of cruelty to animals, and that it was useless to try to counter emotion with logic. He wrote articles in defence of animal experimentation, but relied mainly on winning the support of influential Parliamentarians by appealing to them personally and making sure that they were fully aware of the importance of physiological research.

Paget, Lister, and several other medical men who gave evidence to the Royal Commission, emphasized that in Britain animal experimentation was more carefully controlled by the scientists themselves than it was on the Continent. Burdon-Sanderson was closely questioned about the notorious Handbook. He explained that it was never intended for lay readers. The 'beginners' referred to in the preface were assumed to be trained workers who were new to the authors' departments, but experienced in laboratory procedure. They would be accustomed to using anaesthetics routinely and did not need instruction on this point.

Burdon-Sanderson spoke well, and would have repaired much of the damage caused by the Handbook, but for the evidence given by one of its contributors, Emanuel Klein. Klein, who was Austrian by birth and had received his scientific training in Vienna, came to London in 1871. In 1875 he was a lecturer in histology at St Bartholomew's Hospital, and was also on the staff of the Brown Institute, an organisation carrying out veterinary research. Klein testified that he rarely bothered with anaesthetics when performing animal experiments; in his laboratory they were used only if the animal tried to bite or scratch. He said that the physiologist was usually too preoccupied with the experiment to be concerned about the feelings of the animal. His hearers were so shocked that they questioned him at length, but he did not vary his evidence. Klein dealt the scientist's cause a heavy blow. Although he later said that he had given the wrong impression because of his difficulty with the English language, he could not undo the harm already done.

Legislation was inevitable
After this Paget realized that legislation to control experimentation was inevitable. The Bill that was introduced in May, 1876, would have severely impeded the work of scientists, but its progress through Parliament was delayed. In the meantime the scientists used their influence to have the Bill modified to a form that would be acceptable. Some of them sensed that the Government was losing interest and could perhaps be persuaded to drop the Bill entirely. Paget believed that this was not to be desired; the antivivisection-

ists would reopen their campaign, causing further disruption to the progress of science. He advised his colleagues to press for the early passage of legislation, while making every effort to ensure that it would not be too restrictive. On 22 July a meeting was held between the Home Secretary, Richard Cross and Lord Carnarvon, representing the Government, and Paget, Joseph Hooker, Michael Foster, and Burdon-Sanderson, representing the scientists. As a result of this meeting amendments were made to the Bill that rendered it less obnoxious to the scientists. The Bill was passed in August, 1876.

The Cruelty to Animals Act provided that persons wishing to carry out experiments on live animals had to apply to the Home Secretary for a licence. The application had to be endorsed by the president of one of the eleven scientific and medical bodies in Britain, and by a professor of medicine or another branch of science. The laboratory in which the work was to be carried out also had to be registered. Both the licence and the registration must be renewed annually if the research programme were to continue. The laboratory could be visited at any time by government-appointed inspectors. Experiments without the use of anaesthesia, and experiments using cats, dogs, horses, mules, and asses required additional justification.

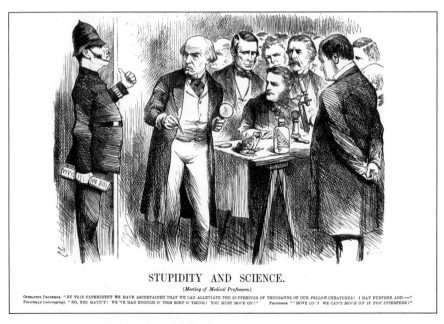

STUPIDITY AND SCIENCE.
(*Meeting of Medical Professors.*)
OPERATING PROFESSOR. " BY THIS EXPERIMENT WE HAVE ASCERTAINED THAT WE CAN ALLEVIATE THE SUFFERINGS OF THOUSANDS OF OUR FELLOW-CREATURES ! I MAY FURTHER ADD—"
POLICEMAN (*interrupting*). " NO, YOU MAYN'T ! WE'VE HAD ENOUGH O' THIS SORT O' THING ! YOU MUST MOVE ON !"   PROFESSOR. "'MOVE ON'? WE CAN'T MOVE ON IF YOU INTERFERE !"

Punch Cartoon on Vivisection, 1876. The four medical men grouped around the table and facing the viewer are, from left, Sir William Jenner, Sir James Paget, Dr Ernest Hart, and Sir William Gull.

As might be expected, the compromise Act did not satisfy either side. Its restrictions hampered the scientists to the extent that a few of them, including Lister, used the laboratories of colleagues in Europe when they wanted to carry out important experiments at short notice. The antivivisectionists thought the Act contained too many loopholes, so they maintained their watch on the scientists. Once again the flames of the controversy died down but were not extinguished.

The Hunterian Oration
On 13 February, 1877, Paget delivered the forty-ninth Hunterian Oration, the greatest of his speeches. John Hunter died in 1793; twenty years later the executors of his will, Sir Everard Home and Dr Matthew Baillie, presented to the Royal College of Surgeons the sum of £1684-4-4d to found an annual oration in their kinsman's honour. They stipulated that it should be 'expressive of the merits in Comparative Anatomy, Physiology, and Surgery, not only of John Hunter, but also of such persons, as should be from time to time deceased, whose labours have contributed to the improvement or extension of Surgical Science.'[14] The Oration was to be held annually on, or close to, John Hunter's birthday, 13 February. Sir Everard Home gave the first Oration in 1814; after 1853 it was made a biennial event. The roll of Hunterian Orators includes many of the great names of nineteenth and twentieth century surgery. (Lister is a notable exception—he was never a Hunterian Orator.)

The Oration of 1877 was fully reported in *The Times,* but a livelier account is contained in the diary of a young man from South Australia. Joseph Verco was a student at St Bartholomew's medical school when he witnessed the events of this wintry afternoon. He trudged through rain and mud along Holborn and turned into Lincoln's Inn Fields:

The old square looked as dark and desolate as usual, with its naked trees and iron railing, and the College itself, with its great pillared portico, was as black as if it was in mourning. It was nearly a quarter to two, though the oration was not to be delivered until three.

A crowd was collected around the very narrow doorway, ready to wait the hour and a quarter rather than miss the treat. Pure surgical gossip was to be heard. 'So poor Sir William has passed away.' 'Yes, he was failing for some months past; he could not manage to get up stairs for some time.' 'Ah yes, shortness of breath pointed to the lungs or kidneys.' 'Ah well, I expect that his practice is already pretty well divided: for you see that a man's patients soon drop off, if he cannot attend to them!' 'Make way for Dr Farre' was shouted out, and a white-haired, very frail old gentleman came along leaning on the arm of a friend, and was allowed to pass through the mob. Evidently the old gynaecologist still knew what was good.

Soon after two, half of the door was unlocked, just enough for one man to squeeze through. What a crush! The poor old G.P.'s began to cry out, in fear of their ribs, demanding that all the doors should be opened; but no sooner were both leaves undone than in they rushed like a flood, very nearly carrying with them the old bald-headed beadle who was standing at the entrance to the hall in his scarlet robe taking the cards. The theatre contained tiers of seats arranged in a semi-circle, and these filled rapidly until there was not even standing room left. Facing the audience was a full-sized copy of Sir Joshua Reynold's portrait of John Hunter, and on a bracket close by a plaster bust of him.

Several of the St Bart's staff were present—Savory and Power in the reserved seats, there was Baker with his arms folded as usual and his monocle in his eye, standing in a corner to see and be seen. There were Willet and Marsh, Cumberbatch, Doran, Walshaw, Keetley, Hart, Hamilton, Rockel, Odell and many others. There was Hope too with his slate pencil-coloured hair plastered down on his head, and his hooked nose. The dear man with his effeminate lisp hardly knew whether to be pleased or to express shame when a blunt jocose surgeon nearby said the question as to whether it were well to sit on the cushion or on bare board was quite a fundamental one. He thought it would be more in his interest to laugh—at any rate he did so. Old Sir William Watson came in midst great applause, as did the old Cock of Guys, Sir William Gull, who looks for all the world like Napoleon Bonaparte: Huxley with his short dark face sat with folded arms and scarce moved a muscle all the while: Tyndal too, with his long old-womany face: Dean Stanley, hair grizzled and cropped short, sharp features and lank form, and the Bishop of London. The Duke of Argyll, whose carrotty hair seemed ready to fly off his head, and the Marquis of Westminster.

After some time in came the macebearer preceding the President, Prescott Hewitt, clad in his robes of office. While he was greeted with thunderous applause, the gold mace was laid on a scarlet cushion before the President, who was supported on his right by the Prince of Wales, and on his left the Duke of Argyll. Close behind came the Hunterian Orator Sir James Paget, who took his place on the dais behind the table bearing the mace, facing President and Prince, and the audience.

Paget's brother from Cambridge was there, as well as his own three sons: all were alike—the same great nose, the prominent eyebrows producing the appearance of a retreating forehead, relieved again by the slightly projecting frontal prominences. The features of the oldest, a barrister, and the second son, a deacon in the Episcopal Church, are sharper than their father, but the youngest is the image of his father—he is to be a surgeon.

As for the oration, that must be eulogised: there is almost no gesture—now his thumb is in his breeches pocket, now his fore-finger is laid almost upon his lips, now in the palm of his left hand, and mostly both of his fists rest on the table as though he were passing an after dinner compliment. His voice did not seem quite as effective as I have known it: in fact he was a little hoarse towards the end of his hour's exertion. His language was very simple: the oration written verbatim would be a specimen of clear, pure English. And very effective. Considering that he had not a single note, simply one or two extracts that he wished to give word for word, the wonder was that the oration was so precise. He has none of the powerful burning eloquence that one would expect in a great public speaker and that one finds more in pulpit perorations: he is very calm and undisturbed in his manner: not unbecoming perhaps in a cool deliberating surgeon, or one who was extolling the memory of such an equable scientific mind as John Hunter. When Paget alluded to the death of Fergusson, he drew tears to the eyes of some of his audience, and time and time again brought down the applause of the house by his felicitous generalisations.[15]

Paget, like many Orators both before and since, chose to speak on John Hunter himself. None could have had a higher regard for the man they were honouring. Paget had devoted a significant part of his working life to the preservation of Hunter's beloved collection of anatomical specimens. He probably felt that he was speaking of an esteemed friend, although Hunter died twenty years before Paget was born.

In the Oration Paget told how it was not until he reached the age of twenty that John Hunter discovered his 'natural fitness for the study of living things'. As a schoolboy he was idle and neglected his studies; in adolescence he still had no plan for the ordering of his life. Almost by chance he left his father's farm in Scotland to work as an assistant to his older brother William, who had made a name for himself in London as a teacher of anatomy. John was put to work dissecting, and preparing specimens to illustrate William's lec-tures. For the first time he experienced the excitement of discover-ing the truth about natural phenomena by combining the skills of his mind, eyes, and hands. It was like being born into a new world:

Hence onward there was no lack of motives. The mind that had been idle, heedless, and aimless had come to its right field of action; every form of intellectual exercise and pleasure was offered to it, and it grew to capacity for all. Gradually the desire of knowledge, both for its own sake and for the happiness of gaining and using it, became like an insatiable passion, a motive to incessant work.[16]

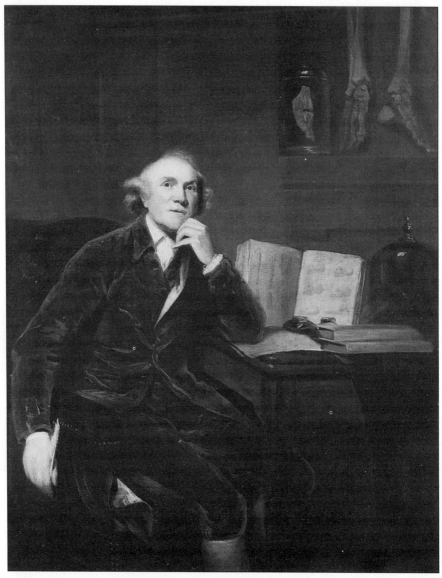

John Hunter. By J Jackson, after Reynolds. (National Portrait Gallery).

Paget described Hunter's joy in the pursuit of truth as being like an athlete's delight in exercising his body. Devising an experiment to solve a problem gave him almost as much satisfaction as the solution itself. His inquiries covered a vast field—human and comparative anatomy, physiology, pathology, and embryology—and in all of these branches of science he made important discoveries. Yet despite his great intellectual capacity he had one deficiency—a difficulty in expressing abstract ideas in words. Thus, when he ventured into a discussion of the 'vital principle of life' he became obscure, although his notes on practical questions are models of clarity. Wisely, he devoted most of his energy to the work he did best:

He may have admired the hypothesis of a vital principle—and he used it wisely—but he much more admired the observation and right use of facts. He collected them as with an avarice; he kept them pure, in memory and manuscript; compared, arranged, and read in them, as he could, the laws of life. Herein was the principal, the best, the most abiding of his works; hence was his great influence in science.[17]

Hunter's great contributions to physiology were not fully appreciated either during his lifetime or for many years after his death. Paget had an explanation for this:

. . . It may well be, that if Hunter had been more apt to teach he would not have been without disciples. Some men by personal influence can make disciples even prematurely. They hasten the unready, attract or compel the unwilling. They are founders of schools before themselves are quite fit to be called scholars. Hunter was utterly void of the qualities by which such teachers make their schools. He had no attractions easy to be felt, no power of persuasion in speech or manner. His lectures were dull, tedious, ill-delivered. He was so busy in his search for knowledge, and so cautious in his estimate of it, that he always delayed to publish what he knew. It was only by the sheer force of his work and example that he could have moved men to follow him. These were enough in surgery and medicine, not enough in the deeper physiology. And thus it was that when he died, poor and with work half done, there was scarcely one who knew how vast and various his labours in this field had been; there was not one who could complete his unfinished essays or the catalogues of his collection. The treasures of his museum and his manuscripts remained unknown for many years. His works had been like waves in advance of the on-coming tide. A few that watched them thought them grand and beautiful; but they broke on the shore in what seemed like only trouble and confusion, and the tide passed over them and hid the treasures they had borne.[18]

His work in pathology had more immediate application to surgery, and was eagerly taken up by the young surgeons who followed him. Thus Abernethy, Astley Cooper, Cline, Home, Lynn, and Blizard all proudly claimed to have been his pupils. They regarded John Hunter as the founder of scientific surgery. Before Hunter, surgeons held a subordinate place in the medical profession; they were even taught their anatomy by physicians.

After the time of Hunter we may trace a well-marked change. Physicians worthily maintained their rank, as they do now; but surgeons rose to it, and in the lessons of Hunter surgery gratefully repaid medicine for the teachings of a century. Following Hunter in the pursuit of science, surgeons soon became the chief anatomists, equal as physiologists and pathologists, and they gained entrance into the ranks of the most educated class. Yes; Hunter did more than anyone to make us gentlemen. And the lesson of this fact is plain and emphatic, for it was not by force of social skill, by money, or any external advantage that he did this. From the few records that we have of him it is clear that he was a rough and simple-mannered man, abrupt and plain in speech, warm-hearted and sometimes rashly generous, emotional and impetuous, quickly moved to tears of sympathy, quickly ablaze with anger and fierce words, never personally attractive, or seeming to have great mental powers, and always far too busy to think of influencing those around him. He had few friends, he gained the personal regard of very few, and no one paid him the homage of mimicry. The vast influence which he exercised on surgery and surgeons was the influence of the scientific mind. What follows? Surely, that if we desire to maintain the rank of gentlemen, to hold this highest prize of our profession, we must do so by the highest scientific culture to which we can attain. And to this we are bound, not for our own advancement alone, but by every motive of the plainest duty.[19]

At the conclusion of the Oration William Gladstone, who was in the audience, was heard to remark, 'Demosthenes himself could not have done better'. This seemed to be the view of all those present. That evening the College held a formal dinner, at which Gladstone was the principal speaker. His address, which lasted for nearly half an hour, included many complimentary references to Paget's career and achievements. Paget's reply took less than a minute:

Mr President, Your Royal Highness, my Lords and Gentlemen—

I have to offer my most heartfelt thanks to Mr Gladstone for the too flattering way in which he has been pleased to speak of me and of my work, and to all of you for the kindness with which his eulogium has been received. There is only one way in which it may be possible for me to surpass Mr Gladstone as an orator, and that way I will proceed to put into practice. You all know that, although speech may be silvern, silence is golden. You shall have the gold![20]

Serjeant Surgeon to Her Majesty Queen Victoria

Sir William Fergusson, whom Paget called 'the greatest master of the art, the greatest practical surgeon of our time', died in February, 1877, three days before the Hunterian Oration. Paget was subsequently appointed Serjeant Surgeon to Her Majesty Queen Victoria, to take Fergusson's place. Stephen Paget spoke of his father's regard for the Royal Family, and his attitude to social distinctions:

. . . He (was) for 41 years a member of the household of Her Majesty Queen Victoria, and for 36 years a member of the household of H.R.H. the Prince of Wales: a very old and very dear servant and friend. He loved to be in his place at the Court, and to be welcome there both for his own sake and for his long record of services. In a letter to his brother, he defines his loyalty as wholly personal and non-political: but it was so far political, in the original meaning of the word, that it was in keeping with that spirit in him which has been described, in a very different context, as *this spirit of order, this hearty acceptance of a place in society, this proud submission which no more desires to rise above its place than it will consent to fall below it.* Wherever he went, he liked to be taken as a surgeon: and if he had chosen any other profession, he would have upheld, with he same steady insistence, the dignity of work and of the professional life, as the thing that places a man.[21]

In 1877 Catherine, the elder daughter of James and Lydia, married the Revd Henry Thompson of Gloucester. The parents took their summer holiday in Gloucester that year, so that they could spend some time with the first of their children to leave the family home.

Paget retires from operating

In 1878 Paget decided that the time had come for him to retire from operating, except for minor cases. Operative surgery had occupied much of his working time for thirty years, but now, at the age of sixty-four, he was beginning to notice in himself signs of the ageing process. The *Vanity Fair* caricature of 1876 shows him as a frail,

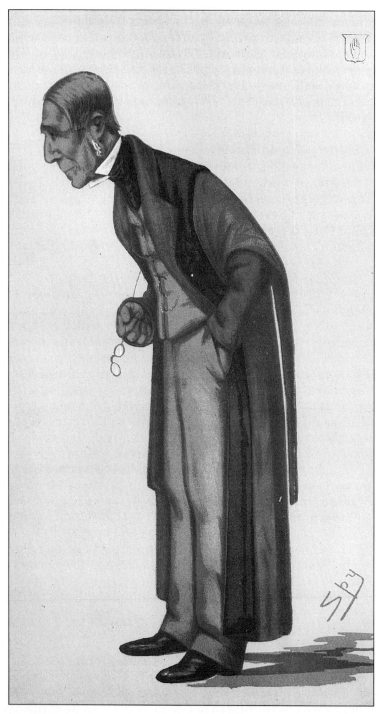

Sir James Paget. Chromolithograph by 'Spy', 1876. (Wellcome Institute).

stooped figure. Although he objected that the drawing was absurdly inaccurate, his thinking may have been influenced by it. There was also the change that was taking place in surgery itself. Some eminent surgeons were still critical of Lister and his antiseptic system, but in practice most of them had incorporated elements of Listerism in their own operating procedures, and in the larger hospitals antiseptic measures were being adopted generally. Thus, William Savory, a leading surgeon on the staff of St Bartholomew's Hospital, attacked Lister at a conference in 1879; but in 1877 Joseph Verco had observed an operation performed at the Hospital under cover of a carbolic spray, and by the time he finished his training there the antiseptic method was being used routinely. With the control of wound infection new and more ambitious operative procedures became possible. If Paget were to continue operating he would need to master new techniques. He decided that it would be wiser to limit himself to the diagnostic practice he found more satisfying, and leave operative surgery to younger men.

President of the Seventh International Congress of Medicine

One of the notable events in nineteenth-century medical history was the Seventh International Congress of Medicine, which took place in August, 1881. When the Sixth Congress was held in Amsterdam in 1878 London was selected as the next venue. The Provisional Committee appointed to plan the London Congress included Sir James Paget, Sir William Jenner, Sir William Gull, Professor Joseph Lister, Sir Prescott Hewitt, and other prominent members of the British medical profession. Paget was elected their President.

The Committee began its work more than two years before the date of the Congress. They intended this to be one of the most important medical conferences ever held, and planned accordingly. They drew up an ambitious scientific programme and invited internationally famous men to head its various sections. They sent out more than 120 000 notices. They also arranged a brilliant social programme, although it was always intended that this would be of secondary importance. The success of the Congress repaid the Committee's efforts. It was attended by over three thousand doctors and scientists, a third of whom were visitors from Europe, the United States, and the colonies. They came to hear and to meet Pasteur, Lister, Virchow, Osler, Charcot, Koch, Huxley, and Darwin. No medical conference before or since could have brought together so many great men.

The Congress was divided into fifteen sections representing various subdivisions of medicine. More than one hundred sectional meetings were held, and some four hundred and fifty scientific papers were presented. There were also many additional informal meetings and discussions. The official languages were English, French, and German, and an interpreter service was provided. The University of London, the Royal College of Physicians, the Royal Academy, the Royal Society, and many other learned bodies made their premises available for meetings and lectures.

The social programme, which was well supported by the visitors and their wives, was given added interest by the patronage of H.R.H. the Prince of Wales and H.I.H. the Crown Prince of Germany. There were receptions and banquets at the Guildhall and the Mansion House. At the Inaugural Meeting on 3 August Paget gave an address of welcome, and at the conclusion of the Congress a week later there was a dinner for twelve hundred guests at the Crystal Palace, followed by a fireworks display.

The British hosts had been aware of possible hostility between their French and German guests; Frenchmen still felt the pain of their country's defeat by Germany in the Franco-Prussian War of 1871. Although it was unlikely that political differences would mar the formal scientific sessions, it was thought advisable to entertain French and German guests at separate functions. There was one happy exception when Lister managed to bring Pasteur and Koch together informally. Koch was telling a small group about his development of solid media that enabled him to obtain pure cultures of micro-organisms, when Lister drew Pasteur into the circle. The patriotic elderly Frenchman listened quietly until Koch had finished speaking; then he held out the hand of friendship to the young German, saying, 'C'est un grand progrès, Monsieur!'[22]

Stephen Paget told how his father's involvement in the Congress temporarily transformed life at Harewood Place:

He kept open house all the week, and three times a day entertained a large party of members of the Congress. The house from morning to night was in a whirl of excitement, but it never lost its feeling of home. The incessant hospitality, the confusion of tongues, the coming and going of all the masters of medicine and surgery with their disciples, the meeting of H.R.H. the Prince of Wales and H.I.H. the Crown Prince of Germany with Darwin, Pasteur, Virchow, Huxley, Tyndall, and other great personages—all these festivities were still 'at home'; he could not easily imagine hospitality anywhere else: and the house, somehow, got through the work.[23]

The Congress left Paget exhausted. He took a short holiday at Chelmsford, but the demands of practice and committee work brought him back to London prematurely. It was probably fatigue that caused him to suffer another severe attack of pneumonia in November. His physician advised him to convalesce in a warmer climate, so as soon as he was fit to travel he set off for Nice, accompanied by his wife and younger daughter, Mary. There he remained for over a month. It was the first time the family were not together for Christmas, but the exchange of many letters and greetings helped to compensate for the separation.

The depression that so often afflicted Paget during an illness soon lifted; the letters he wrote from Nice convey the joy of returning health in pleasurable surroundings, although one that he wrote to Catherine shortly before returning home is in a more contemplative mood:

> To Stephen, 13 December— . . . The open windows, and the hot sunshine pouring in—too hot to sit in it—and the Mediterranean, bright blue in front of us, and so clear that, as its waves roll in, one sees right through their curves and they look quite transparent and jade-coloured. And I have carnations from our little garden in my button-hole; and our bouquet at breakfast, bought for half a franc, had abundant roses and violets and orange-flowers. I am half-inclined to say nothing about it, for it is enough to make you unhappily envious in hearing of it: but it shall be an additional reason for making me wish you to have, after May, the jolliest holiday in your life. *Temp.* (not mine, but of our balcony at 11 a.m.) 68 to 70 degrees.[24]

> To Catherine, 11 January— . . . I do not forget that I am growing old, and am already much older than it used to seem at all likely that I should ever be: and with increasing years one's power of recovery from illness becomes less complete; but I should be very grateful, and try to be, for the great gain which I have had here. Still, it is nearly time to be home: the great happiness you all wish me is there: especially, the happiness of being near you all, and so more consciously one among you all.[25]

Although his immediate recovery was satisfactory, this illness seemed to mark the beginning of Paget's descent into old age.

Chapter 8

The Committee Man

The International Medical Congress revived the vivisection controversy. British delegates used the Congress platform to voice their
indignation at the Act of 1876, and their comments were given wide
publicity in the daily newspapers. The antivivisectionists mounted
a counter-attack. Frances Cobbe and her fellow members of the
Victoria Street Society perused the Congress *Proceedings,* checking
the reports of animal experiments against the Home Office records
of licences issued. To their delight, they found what appeared to
be a glaring breach of the Act by Dr David Ferrier, a neuro-
physiologist.

The trial of Dr David Ferrier
Ferrier was a member of the medical staff of King's College Hospital, London, where he was carrying out important research on the
localization of function in the brain. He demonstrated that, despite
the seemingly random pattern of convolutions on the surface of the
brain, it was possible to define very precisely the areas that control
various sensory and motor functions. The old, imaginative concepts
of phrenology were at last being discredited.

Ferrier's work was given added impetus by Lister's success in
controlling infection. The surgical removal of tumours of the brain
was now practicable, provided the site of the tumour could be
determined pre-operatively. In 1876 Ferrier published a book, *The
Functions of the Brain,* which attracted considerable attention. At
the Congress a large audience gathered to hear him describe his
experiments on monkeys. He told how he removed small segments
of the animals' brains, allowed them to recover from the surgery,
and then studied their residual disabilities. He found that he could
reproduce at will patterns of disability matching those seen in
human patients suffering from various diseases of the brain. Thus
he could relate each disability, or 'neurological defect' to a corresponding region of the brain. With this knowledge the location of a
tumour of the human brain could be deduced. Other workers had
attempted something of the kind, but because they used lower
orders of animals their results were not so readily related to human
disease states.

Some of the monkeys Ferrier had used in his experiments were
displayed at the Congress and were available for members of the
audience to examine. The doctors who saw them realized that they
were witnessing the beginning of a new phase of medical progress.

(Indeed, three years later the first surgical removal of a brain tumour, which had been localized by the application of Ferrier's principles, was carried out.) But to the antivivisectionists the monkeys displayed at the Congress appeared only as the pathetic victims of man's cruelty and ambition. When they found that Ferrier had not applied for a licence to perform his experiments they demanded that he be brought to trial.

The medical profession rallied behind Ferrier; the British Medical Association offered to pay his legal expenses. In his defence Ferrier stated that, although he had devised and supervised the experiments, he had not himself performed the operations on the monkeys; this work was done by a colleague in his laboratory, GF Yeo, and Yeo had obtained the appropriate licence. Ferrier was acquitted.

The episode profoundly disturbed both factions. It convinced the antivivisectionists that the Act was so easily circumvented as to be useless. It demonstrated to the scientists their need for an organization as effective as that of their opponents, to protect them from harassment and to promote scientific research. The inaugural meeting of the Association for the Advancement of Medicine by Research was held at the Royal College of Physicians in May, 1882. The College President, Sir William Gull, was elected the Association's first President; Sir James Paget was Vice-President. Members of the Council were Lister, Burdon-Sanderson, Foster, and Yeo. At first the policy of the AAMR was to attempt to win popular support by the publication of pamphlets explaining the importance of the work of the biological scientists. A year later they decided that they could achieve more by working behind the scenes. The Association offered the services of its Council to the Home Secretary, to assist him in the evaluation of licence applications. The acceptance of the offer meant that the Association was able to influence the administration of the Act. Although the arrangement was quite irregular, the Association does not appear to have abused its privilege. It produced information leaflets for the guidance of licence applicants, and recommended the rejection of a number of unsatisfactory applications. The antivivisectionists objected to the arrangement, but were unable to stir the public into supporting any action against it. Peace returned for nearly thirty years.

At the height of the public debate on the trial of Ferrier, Paget contributed an article to the journal *Nineteenth Century*. He drew attention to the pain inflicted on animals for the pleasure of sportsmen, and for human adornment, yet these practices passed unchallenged. He continued:

At the present time 20 000 persons are annually killed by venomous snakes in India. If the discovery of a remedy without experiments on animals would come later by, say, five years, than one made with their help, would it be nothing to have lost 100 000 lives? The case is worth considering because of an almost absurd consequence of the Vivisection Act. I may pay a rat-catcher to destroy all the rats in my house with any poison that he pleases; but I may not myself, unless with a licence from the Home Secretary, poison them with snake-poison, nor, without an additional certificate, try to keep them alive after it.[1]

But most of his work in support of experimental science was done quietly through contact, or through the AAMR. He was still Vice-President of this organization in 1892, when he wrote to one of his sons, probably Stephen:

I hope you will not think that I am beginning to love publicity because my name has lately been appearing in the newspapers. I have let it do so as seldom and as gently as I could: but it was impossible for me among many friends to appear indifferent to the vivisection-question which some of the clergy, chiefly Bishop Barry, were so foolish as to raise. It will be quiet, I hope, now for some time: certainly I shall be; and I can safely plead that I am too old for controversies and am happy in hating them more than ever.[2]

Stephen Paget was himself later involved in the antivivisection dispute. He became the secretary of the AAMR and wrote extensively in defence of animal experimentation.

Continuing contributions to medicine
In 1882 Paget reported seven new cases of *osteitis deformans*. They resembled his first series very closely, except that none had been observed to develop cancer. A specimen of bone from one of the new cases was examined under the microscope by Henry Butlin; the appearance was identical to that reported by him in 1876. Thus Paget's disease of bone was confirmed as a disease entity.

The following year, 1883, he was elected Vice-Chancellor of the University of London, in succession to Sir George Jessel, who died earlier in the year. Although Paget was not himself a university graduate, he occupied this important position with distinction for twelve years. Sir Joshua Fitch, a member of the University Senate, later recalled the striking contrast between the personalities of Paget and his predecessor. Jessel had the reputation of being one of the strongest men on the Equity bench; his chairmanship of the Senate was equally decisive. Paget, on the other hand, preferred to arrive at important decisions by consensus. When this was not possible he would seek a compromise, or would defer discussion of a divisive matter to allow emotions to cool. Both types of leadership have their merits and deficiencies. It often happens, as in this case, that successive elected leaders are of opposite types.

Paget attended the Eighth International Congress of Medicine held in Copenhagen in 1884. He enjoyed it, although the Danes provided such lavish hospitality that the scientific programme was rather overshadowed. From Copenhagen he embarked on an extensive holiday tour that took him across Germany to St Petersburg, Moscow, Kiev, and Warsaw, then home via Dresden and Berlin. He was probably accompanied by his wife and several friends, although his letters do not identify the members of the party. The three days they spent in St Petersburg were crammed with visits to churches and art galleries, as well as meeting with old friends from home. Then they went on to Moscow. Comparisons with St Petersburg were inevitable:

> Everything great or rare or interesting at St Petersburg is surpassed here, if the splendid picture-gallery and the collection of Greek ornaments and statuettes be excepted—certainly a grander gallery than any I have seen, richer in Raphaels, Rembrandts, Van Dycks, and nearly every Flemish artist's work, than I could have guessed at. But leaving all these, all the wonders at St Petersburg are here surpassed. The splendour of the Churches, the glare of their decorations, the pious customs of the people, the shabby miserable looks, the seeming utter poverty and idleness of many of them, are more than one can describe. But really, the place is past describing. The Kremlin, of which one had a vague notion as of a huge Mosque, is, in fact, a vast space enclosed with turreted and towered walls, like a fortress, nearly two miles in circumference and containing three or more palaces, about 6 Churches, 3 convents, and a great review-ground, and I have not yet seen what besides. Among the churches are some of the most gorgeous—as one enters such an one, it seems within all gold; for the walls and pillars and roofs are nearly all covered with gorgeous Icons, altars, banners, lamps and whatever else may look glorious and costly. And of these, less or more grand, there are in Moscow more than 350. Yet the priests are among the least cleanly of the people; none, it is said, respect them; none are taught by them; they are a separate class, mingling with neither higher nor lower. And with all the apparent wealth of the Churches the town in most places looks utterly dirty, ill-paved, unswept; and the majority of the people match well with it. I have never seen contrasts so awful: and the contrast is the more marked because of the rarity of anything that might seem midway between the extremes of grandeur and of misery.[3]

The following year, 1885, was one in which honours were conferred on both James and George Paget. In March James received a telegraph from Charcot, informing him that he had been elected a Corresponding Member of the Académie des Sciences. Pasteur's congratulatory letter, which shortly followed, was an expression of friendship rather than a social formality. In a letter to one of his sons Paget referred to the honour as 'the highest distinction of its kind, the "blue riband" of science; far more honourable than anything I should have thought that I had fairly earned. I must try to be harmlessly proud of it.'[4]

In December, 1885, George Paget was made a Knight Commander of the Order of the Bath, in recognition of his services to medicine. He had retired from the post of physician to Addenbrooke's Hospital, Cambridge, after serving that hospital for forty-five years. Sir George, although not a prolific writer for the scientific journals, had become known for his efforts to improve standards of medical training and practice. He had been instrumental in having tests of practical skills included in the examinations taken by medical undergraduates at Cambridge, thereby setting an example that other examining bodies later followed. One of George's sons, Dr Charles Paget, was for several years James's assistant and secretary.

It was also in 1885 that James completed a second edition of the catalogue of the museum of the Royal College of Surgeons. The first edition had been seven years in the making; the second took just as long. During the forty years that the first catalogue had been in use several thousand new specimens had been added. These were listed in supplements, but in 1878 the Council decreed that a new catalogue should be compiled. Sir James Paget was appointed to supervise the work, with the assistance of Dr Goodhart and Mr Alban Doran. The first volume of the new edition appeared in 1881, the fourth and last volume in 1885. Goodhart described how the work was carried out:

We used to meet at two o'clock on Saturday afternoons, sometimes on other days, in the Museum galleries, and go over the new specimens together. Sir James would take the preparation, and one of us would read the description of the specimen. I can see him now, as it were but yesterday, with his eyes intent on the jar before him, listening, and always insisting that the description should point out all that could be seen, and nothing more: but the description of all that the specimen showed had to be as complete as possible. He was very particular about the style; but I think this came out more in the corrections that I noticed afterwards in the copy or proof than in the criticisms that he made at the time. I always thought that he was too careful of the feelings of his assistants, though very fond of his child 'the original catalogue' and very determined that nothing should be added therein that did not conform to the standard he had originally set up, and which time has proved to be a worthy model. The amount Sir James did was by far the larger part. Looking back upon it from this distance of time, it almost seems that I did very little: and, quite early in the work, he astonished as well as delighted us by voluntarily undertaking all the arrangement of headings, references, cross-references, and indices; because, as he said, it had always been a pleasure to him to make an index. 'Verify your references,' was another maxim he often used. To most men, I think it might be said, making a catalogue of specimens is not an interesting occupation: but Sir James so beguiled the time with stories and talk that those Saturday afternoons have often come back to me with fragrant memories, so keen was the enjoyment that he inspired.[5]

When the last volume was published the College, as a mark of its appreciation, commissioned the sculptor Sir Edgar Boehm to make a marble bust of Paget.

In 1886 Paget finished another writing task. The memoirs, on which he had been working for five years, were brought to a close and placed in the care of his son Stephen. He then turned his attention to the vast collection of notes on the cases he had seen since his earliest days in practice. He had always believed, and taught, that every medical practitioner should try to improve his personal skill and also contribute to the general body of scientific knowledge by reviewing his own experience. In accordance with this belief he had amassed notes on thousands of cases. The information had been recorded; it now remained for him to analyse it and extract its lessons. This task occupied most of his evenings at home for the next five years, a period in which his practice was declining. Instead of having between twenty and thirty letters to write to referring doctors at the end of each day's consulting, he now had only five or six. Younger men who had once been his students were now themselves established consultants, while many of his own generation were retiring from practice. But those colleagues and old patients who still valued his opinion above all others were sufficiently numerous to give him all the work he desired.

The Pasteur Committee
Another committee was soon to occupy his time and thoughts. Several years previously, Pasteur had shown that it was possible to extract from the spinal cord of an animal that had died of rabies a substance that, if injected into a healthy animal, prevented the recipient from contracting the disease. Even an animal that had

already been infected with the rabies micro-organism could be protected, provided the treatment was begun soon enough. In 1885 Pasteur used his treatment for the first time on human subjects who had been bitten by rabid dogs. His results were so impressive that government authorities, as well as the scientific community, became interested.

In England, Mr Joseph Chamberlain, President of the Local Government Board, established the Pasteur Committee to investigate and report on Pasteur's claims. The eight-member Committee had Sir James Paget as its Chairman, Mr Victor Horsley as Secretary. Horsley was a young surgeon who carried out research in physiology. At its first meeting, held on 15 April 1886, the Committee decided to send three of its members, one of them Horsley, to observe the work on rabies being done in Pasteur's laboratories.

When Horsley's party arrived in Paris they found Pasteur anxiously pre-occupied with a group of patients who were in a desperate plight, having been attacked by a rabid dog some days previously. The Englishmen were left in no doubt that their visit was inopportune. But a letter from Paget, which Pasteur received the next day, seemed to change their situation completely. Thereafter Horsley's party received every assistance.

They began their visit with open minds, but were soon convinced of the effectiveness of Pasteur's method of preventing rabies. Horsley brought back with him two rabbits that had been infected with the rabies virus; using material obtained from these, he repeated Pasteur's work and confirmed his results. The Committee's report, compiled by Paget and Horsley, stated that the claims made by Pasteur for his treatment were verified. But the Committee recommended that efforts should be concentrated on eradication of the disease, rather than on the treatment of victims. An island nation like Britain had the advantage of being able to quarantine all dogs brought into the country. This measure, combined with the extermination of stray dogs, would result in the elimination of rabies from Britain within three years. The Committee's advice was accepted, and proved to be sound.

The sharing of work for the Pasteur Committee enabled Paget and Horsley to become well acquainted. Horsley was then barely thirty years old, but he had already made a name for himself with his original work on the thyroid gland. His interests had then turned to neuro-physiology and neuro-surgery. During the year that he served on the Pasteur Committee he was appointed surgeon to the National Hospital for Nervous Diseases, and was elected to the Fellowship of the Royal Society. Horsley was by nature a reformer. A strict teetotaller and non-smoker, he campaigned against the consumption of alcohol and tobacco with a zeal that was almost fanatical. Paget could be tolerant of quite significant

weaknesses in men who had earned his respect in other ways, but
he found it difficult to forgive eccentricity, the deliberate adoption
of bizarre manners or attitudes. Stephen Paget describes one of the
very rare occasions on which his father caused a guest some
embarrassment:

> ... Of all the younger men (Horsley) was the one whose work my
> father most admired, saying of some of it that it marked an epoch
> in the history of medicine; but I remember him dining at my
> father's house in 1887: of course he took neither wine, nor a
> cigarette after dinner, and my father looked across the table at
> him, with affection just touched with resentment of the unusual,
> and said 'Haven't you *one* vice?' Horsley laughed and blushed,
> and said, 'I'm afraid I've got a great many, Sir James'[6]

Smallpox and vaccination

Two years later another public health problem was proving so
difficult to solve that the Government decided on a Royal Commission. The first recorded epidemic of smallpox occurred in Syria in
the fourth century. In the Middle Ages the disease spread across
Europe and reached Britain. In the second half of the seventeenth
century there were several smallpox epidemics in England; the
disease then waned, but did not die out. In eighteenth century
England, with its population of eight million, there was an average
of two thousand deaths per year from smallpox, but when epidemics
broke out the death rate soared to many times this figure. Half of
those who contracted the disease died, and those who survived were
permanently scarred. The spread of smallpox was not related to
poverty or insanitary living conditions; there were as many pock-
marked faces in London's drawing-rooms as there were in the
taverns. All sections of society feared the disease, and all were eager
to learn of anything that could protect them from it.

The first step towards this end was the work of a remarkable
woman. Lady Mary Wortley Montagu returned to England in 1718
after spending two years in Turkey, where her husband was the
British ambassador. There she had observed the practice of
inoculation against smallpox. Fluid from a smallpox blister was
injected into the skin of a healthy person; this usually resulted in a
very mild attack of smallpox that gave lasting immunity to the
disease. Lady Mary succeeded in popularizing inoculation, but with
experience its risks became apparent. It sometimes actually caused
severe smallpox and could start epidemics of the disease. Thus Dr
Edward Jenner met with an enthusiastic response when, in 1798,
he described a new method of acquiring immunity.

While working in his country practice in Gloucester, Jenner observed that cattle suffered from a disease known as cowpox, which

was readily transmitted to humans. It produced blisters resembling those of the early stages of smallpox, but it was a mild affliction that soon resolved. When country people told Jenner that milkmaids who had had cowpox seemed to be immune to smallpox, he wondered if this immunity could be deliberately induced. He decided to follow the dictum of his old master, John Hunter, and solve the problem by means of an experiment. This experiment was to become famous. In May 1796 Sarah Nelmes, a milkmaid at a neighbouring Gloucester farm, developed cowpox blisters on her hands. Jenner took some of the fluid, or lymph, from Sarah's blisters and injected it into the skin of James Phipps, a healthy eight-year-old boy. The boy developed typical cowpox blisters, which soon healed, and a week later he was perfectly well again. In July Jenner injected James with smallpox. It had no effect—the boy had been successfully immunized. This process became known as 'vaccination', from the Latin *vacca*—a cow. The lymph could be obtained directly from a cow, but in urban areas it was more convenient to use the arm-to-arm method, in which lymph was obtained from the blister on the arm of one vaccinated person to inject into others.

Vaccination brought into disrepute
There was soon a brisk demand for vaccination. Unfortunately, many ill-informed or dishonest vaccinators did not follow the correct procedure. Careless use of the arm-to-arm method sometimes resulted in inadvertent inoculation with true smallpox, or with other skin infections. Injudicious vaccination of sickly infants caused some infant deaths. These failures tended to bring the process into disrepute. There were also people who objected to vaccination on religious grounds; some argued that smallpox epidemics were the will of God, others questioned the morality of injecting animal substance into humans. Nevertheless, it could not be denied that smallpox epidemics by-passed communities in which there was a high incidence of vaccination.

In 1808 Parliament voted that vaccination should be given free of charge to all who would accept it, but less than half the population took advantage of the offer. The Poor Law of 1834 placed groups of parishes under the direction of Boards of Governors who, in addition to administering other provisions of the Poor Law, were to encourage their people to be vaccinated. In 1853 vaccination of infants was made compulsory; parents who failed to comply were liable to pay a fine of twenty shillings. The fine could be imposed repeatedly, as long as the offenders remained obdurate. But the law was not rigorously enforced, and in some regions as many as one third of infants escaped vaccination. The Franco-Prussian War of 1870–71 brought an influx of French refugees, and a serious epidemic soon followed. This resulted in stricter enforcement of the law, and renewed protests from the objectors. Some still feared that vaccination could cause other diseases as serious as the one it prevented. To fine parents who believed they were acting in their children's best interests seemed undemocratic.

Paget sits on Royal Commission

The task of the Royal Commission was to review all the relevant evidence and points of view, to determine whether vaccination was both safe and effective, and to advise on whether or not it should continue to be compulsory. There were fifteen Commissioners, with Lord Herschell as their Chairman. Prominent medical men who were members were Sir James Paget, Sir William Savory, Sir Michael Foster, and Mr Jonathan Hutchinson. The Commission had its first meeting in May 1889, and did not complete its work until the final report was submitted in August 1896. It met on 136 occasions, and took evidence from 187 witnesses; it investigated claims and reports from every part of the country. Three of the Commissioners (one of them Sir William Savory) died during this time. Paget, who was eighty-two when the Commission completed its work, took the chair for thirty-nine of its last forty meetings. Despite his great age he was, according to Jonathan Hutchinson, a very useful member:

> He was regular and punctual on all occasions, and no one whom I have ever known could express his views more clearly or tersely, or make more sure of their effect. Many a discussion which threatened to be interminable was concluded by a few chosen words from his lips. He did not speak often, and never lengthily, nor did he ever take up much of the time of the Commission in cross-questioning the witnesses. He was always a most attentive listener, and if ever a question of his own was interposed, it went to the heart of the matter. . . . The extent to which he had made himself familiar with vaccination-literature was wonderful, and he never quoted facts inaccurately.[7]

The Commission concluded that vaccination was the only effective method of preventing smallpox. They found that, if properly performed, it was safe. Claims that tuberculosis, leprosy, and cancer had been transmitted by vaccination could not be substantiated, but even so, the Commission recommended that arm-to-arm vaccination should cease. Glycerinated calf lymph should be the only material used, as this had been shown to be free of any organisms other than the cowpox virus.

The Commission recommended that all infants should be vaccinated before the age of six months, and that the process should be repeated at the age of twelve years, since experience had shown that immunity gradually waned during childhood. Paget believed in universal vaccination, but he disagreed with its being made compulsory. He thought some people so resented compulsion that, for this reason alone, they would avoid having their children vaccinated. When Lord Herschell proposed that the Commission's report should include a recommendation that the rights of conscientious objectors be recognized, Paget supported him against strong opposition. The recommendation was included in the Commission's report.

Shortly after the Commission submitted its final report, and while the Government was still considering its Vaccination Act Amendments Bill, there were serious epidemics of smallpox in Gloucester (Jenner's own county) and Yorkshire. In both counties there were a number of parishes whose Guardians had been lax in enforcing the vaccination of infants, with the result that a high proportion of the population had no immunity. The mortality in these parishes, as compared with others in which there was a high rate of compliance with the law, provided a telling argument in favour of universal vaccination.

These events fuelled the fires of controversy. Arthur Wollaston Hutton, an eloquent opponent of vaccination, wrote a book entitled *The Vaccination Question*, which he introduced with the comment:

At a select social club in the West-end of London vaccination is, I am told, one of four subjects (the other three being politics, religion, and Wagner) which members are forbidden to discuss, on the grounds that such discussion leads nowhere, and only ends in irritation.[8]

The Government included most of the Commission's recommendations in its Vaccination Bill, but the conscience clause met with strong opposition and almost caused the Bill to be abandoned. When the Bill reached the House of Lords, Lister, who had been raised to the peerage in 1897, spoke in favour of the conscience clause. Like Paget, he believed in universal vaccination, but thought that attempts at more rigid enforcement would be self-defeating. The Bill finally became an Act with the conscience clause intact. Some regarded the inclusion of the clause as a victory for wisdom and democracy, while others maintained with equal vigour that it made the Act ineffectual. Both sides of the debate would have been gratified to know that, less than a century later, smallpox would be totally eliminated, not only from Britain, but from the whole world, by the efficient use of vaccination.

Paget sometimes too ready to compromise?

Some people thrive on dissension; it stimulates them to greater effort and lifts them to heights of achievement that they would otherwise never contemplate. Paget was not one of these. He abhorred heated argument, whether it occurred between individuals, or between the supporters of reform movements and their opponents. If attacked when he believed himself to be in the right, he would stand his ground doggedly, for as long as it took to exhaust his adversary, but he would not strike the first blow and was always glad to end the conflict and shake hands.

In the early part of his career he had been able to avoid becoming involved in medical politics. His triumph over the hospital-apprenticeship system and his reform of the St Bartholomew's medical school were achieved peaceably, with hard work and determination. He believed that reform should be brought about gradually, by the efforts of well-disposed individuals, rather than by organized movements with their unfortunate tendency to destroy the good along with the bad.

In his mature years Paget's professional standing led to his being appointed to the administrative bodies of a number of academic institutions and learned societies. These appointments necessarily involved him in medical politics and required him to take sides in some controversial issues. He found this distasteful, particularly when his views differed from those of men he respected and whose advice he sought on other matters. Perhaps it was his natural modesty that made him too ready to think, when in this situation, that he himself must be wrong. It was only in this role as an administrator that any criticism was ever levelled at Paget. Thus, a fellow member of the Council of the Royal College of Surgeons wrote:

> Paget's management of other men and of affairs was very skilful, and depended to a great extent upon his constant willingness to listen to argument and to reconsider his opinions. No one could yield to adverse pressure with a better grace, and he never seemed to be so possessed by an idea as not to be able to throw it aside. Perhaps he was rather too fond of compromise, and he has been known to express wonder how men could so easily persuade themselves that their own views must of necessity be correct. In the Council of the College of Surgeons he exercised great influence, which was partly due to his inclination to be with the majority. He went with the tide to a considerable extent, and would seldom persevere in an opposition which seemed unlikely to be successful; not from the slightest inclination towards timeserving, but from genuine intellectual modesty, which led him to distrust his own judgement, and to think of the probability that

others might understand the question at issue better than he did himself.[9]

Dr Pye-Smith, who served on the Senate of London University during Paget's Vice-Chancellorship, wrote:

> ... He appeared sometimes to carry his admirable gentleness, his *mitis sapientia,* to excess. He could not bear to say a word that might inflict even the most trivial annoyance on those who were most careless of it themselves. One occasion illustrated this weakness, if such it were. On a committee of the Senate, it had long been felt that some change in certain official positions was necessary, and after due conference it was agreed that a member of the Committee should when the time came propose the change generally desired. The proposal was duly made as arranged beforehand, and all looked to Sir James to support it. But he kept his eyes fixed on the papers before him, and made no sign: there was nothing to be said, but it was felt that on that occasion unwillingness to give pain had been carried as far as possible without merging into weakness.[10]

These comments were contained in eulogies written shortly after Paget's death; under different circumstances the writers may have been more outspoken.

Women in medicine
Paget's attitude to women in the medical profession typifies his response to reform, particularly reform that evoked strong and irrational emotions. He was kind and helpful to Dr Elizabeth Blackwell when she visited St Bartholomew's Hospital in 1850, although he was clearly not in sympathy with her later efforts to promote 'female doctordom'. Elizabeth Garrett, the first woman to obtain an English medical qualification, began practising in London in 1867, knowing that many of her male colleagues would be glad to see her starve. But no doctor can practise in isolation from the rest of the profession; Dr Garrett needed to be able to call on the assistance of consultants for special cases. One of her first requests for help was made to James Paget. He responded promptly, gave her expert advice, and remained her friend thereafter. It is significant that before they met Paget these two women had both successfully overcome many obstacles in order to obtain their qualifications; they could not be regarded as mere notoriety-seekers.

The case of Miss Ellen Colborne was different. This young woman hoped to begin medical training by attending the lectures of Dr Black and Mr Savory at St Bartholomew's Hospital. Her application and fees for the 1865 course were accepted. But when she tried to attend Dr Black's first lecture the male students created an uproar, hissing, booing, and stamping their feet until she left the room. Her appearance at Mr Savory's class prompted the lecturer to ask the students whether they wished him to proceed. All but one voted against his delivering the lecture in the presence of a female. Miss Colborne was not heard of again at the Hospital. (Female students were not admitted to St Bartholomew's until 1947 !)

The story of Ellen Colborne is told in Henry Butlin's diary of his student years.[11] Butlin does not mention Paget in his account of the episode, nor does Paget refer to Miss Colborne in his memoirs, although it seems unlikely that he was unaware of her plight. Paget was held in such high esteem at the Hospital that he could perhaps have softened the students' attitude, just as he had persuaded the class of 1850 to accept Elizabeth Blackwell. But the circumstances surrounding the presence of the two women at the Hospital were different. Firstly, Ellen Colborne's academic ability was unproved and, secondly, the climate of opinion had turned much more strongly against women in medicine during the fifteen-year interval. In 1850 the idea of a significant number of women entering the profession seemed to be not worth taking seriously; in 1865 many men took it very seriously indeed, and opposed it vehemently. The reasons they usually advanced—women's supposed lack of physical and mental stamina, and the indelicacy of teaching anatomy and physiology to mixed classes—were too trivial to explain their strength of feeling. The real reasons were much more fundamental; male pride and male pockets were being attacked. If the 'weaker' sex showed that they, too, could be good doctors, male superiority would be undermined. Furthermore, in the average practice half the patients were women, many of whom would probably have preferred a medical adviser of their own sex. Thus female competitors threatened the incomes of their male colleagues, at a time when many young doctors were struggling to survive.

During the preparations for the International Congress of 1881, Paget had to decide whether to support or oppose the admission of women doctors as delegates. He expressed his views in a letter to Sir Joseph Hooker:

> I think that I am of just the same opinion as yourself in regard to the admission of women to the profession and to the Congress. But while we and some more are 'on the whole' and 'rather lukewarmly' in favour of their admission, there is a very much larger number who are so altogether and hotly against it that in any meeting they would carry their opinions by a very large majority and a very loud one too. Their objections are, I believe, chiefly sentimental: but I cannot help feeling that their sentiment 'against' is so very much stronger than my reasons 'for', that the

sentiment may, in a question of this kind, have a right to prevail over the reason.

I may confess, too, that I am influenced towards a negative posture in this case by what I have heard of some of the American and Zurich women-doctors, whom it would be difficult to exclude though few decent Englishmen would like to be associated with them. Let me add that the 'legal qualification' does not give legal right to be a member of a voluntary association. No doubt there will, in any case, be a row: but the row in the event of exclusion will, I can assure you, be far less than it would be in that of admission.[12]

Rather than take the slightest risk of having the Congress marred by disputation, Paget was prepared to exclude all women. A century later this action seems unreasonable and ungenerous. Even if some of the women doctors were not perfect ladies, by Paget's own account many of the male members of the profession could not be classed as gentlemen. In any case, the total number of women doctors was so small that there would probably have been only a handful of them at the Congress. But they had to be debarred lest their mere presence should enrage some of the men. Exclusion from the brilliantly successful event would not, in the long term, have been a further hindrance to the careers of the women concerned, since they would have access to all the papers when the Proceedings were published a few months later. But some of them must have been wounded by this affront to their hard-won professional status.

James Paget's wife and his mother, as well as his two daughters, were intelligent, thoughtful women, who evidently found fulfilment in woman's traditional domestic role. They gave him no reason to believe that other women had different needs and aspirations. Yet Stephen Paget later spoke of his Aunt Kate, who never married, as being like a caged eagle, beating her wings against the conventions that confined her to her cottage, with its daily round of petty tasks. If James Paget did not understand his sister, he was no less perceptive than most otherwise enlightened men of his generation.

Thus Paget's attitude to the prevailing social system seems to have been ambivalent. He willingly extended the helping hand to individuals who were struggling to rise above the plane to which they were born; but he believed that a man should accept the challenge of life, and not expect the social system to be changed to meet his needs. Canon Scott Holland, who was a contemporary of James Paget's sons, and a frequent guest at Harewood Place, thought that Paget's outlook was a product of the age in which he lived, an age that ended with the close of the nineteenth century:

This brave and healthy belief of Sir James in a man's power to make his way through the facts as they are, is, after all, however humane and tender-hearted and pitiful he himself was, a gospel for the strong; and it is the weak of whom we have especially learned to think . . . Sir James belonged to the earlier day, when the best men believed that it was a man's own fault if he could not make something of life; and when, therefore, each had, for his main duty, to do his own bit with all his might. Now, the world's great trouble has cast its shadow on us all. We are all driven to take our share in its burden and in its undoing. To decline this, now that it has once been felt and faced, would be the work of the 'bad citizen.'[13]

But Scott Holland spoke as one of the leaders of the Christian Social Union, a group who were working for sweeping reforms of the social system. Charles Newman, author of *The Evolution of Medical Education in the Nineteenth Century,* believed that men of Paget's outlook are to be found in any age. Paget could have been the prototype for Newman's 'internal reformers':

Reform in medical education, like reform in any activity, is of two kinds. Those concerned may spontaneously improve things, putting their own house in order, on a basis of reason and in a quiet, slow pedestrian way, a process of internal reform. Or more conscious reformers may grapple with improvement in fields outside their immediate personal concern, correcting the faults of others, under an emotional stimulus, by the exciting, large-scale processes of agitation and legal reform. This is the process of external reform. Some people prefer one, some the other. To the internal reformer, external reform is an aspect of the romantic spirit, disturbing, dangerous, revolutionary, and in all ways undesirable. To the external reformer, the slow evolutionary process of internal reform is an irritating tinkering with manifest inefficiency, a waste of time, and a truckling to vested interest. The two types of people are fundamentally different psychologically and the twain never meet.[14]

Chapter 9

The Work is Finished

Paget observed the ageing process in himself with as much detachment as if he were studying a tree in his garden. He was seventy-two years old when he concluded his memoirs with a description of old age:

> It is very difficult for an old man—say for one who is 70, and not unhealthy—to observe all the changes which in the passing years are in progress in him. Even in many things which he can see and feel, and which are certainly changing in him, he may be unable to discern the change. No man over 70 walks with the same pliant, elastic, easy step as he walked at 30 or 40; but many, over 70, I think are not conscious of the change: they can see it in others, they cannot feel it in themselves. Anyone, I suppose, could discern the difference in voice and speech of a friend over 70, while he remembers what it was 20 or 30 years before; but to the old man himself, I suspect, the change is often imperceptible. He does not observe the diminished range of notes, or the veiled sound of his s, or, worse still, its shrill whistle. It is only when he puts these and the like things to a careful test that he finds the change. He may find it by timing his walk—his full speed may be half-a-mile less in the hour; or by trying his voice—he cannot reach his former highest or lowest notes, or sustain any note so long as once he could. And so it is throughout: the change has been so gradual, that it is only with care that even the accumulated contrast can be discerned. With such care, the changes can be seen, and so can the reasonableness of the diminution of practice. Herein is one of the many things in which the old need education as much as the young do: they need self-examination, self-teaching. The 'I will' is, in many of their designs, slow and hesitating and procrastinating. Their word should be 'I will now,' and the work should follow instantly.[1]

Paget himself never lacked the will to work. Although his practice diminished to the extent that he saw only an occasional patient, he was still mentally energetic. He played an important part in the Royal Commission on Vaccination, and contributed to the work of other scientific and charitable organisations, at an age when many men are unable to bear responsibility.

Age did, however, make him even less inclined to become involved in disputes in which no important scientific or humanitarian principle was a stake. Thus in his old age he found himself out of sympathy with his friend Florence Nightingale, when she bitterly opposed the standardisation of nursing qualifications and the establishment of a register of qualified nurses. The British Nurses' Association, which had been founded in 1887, believed that without these measures nursing would not be recognised as a profession. About half the nursing body supported this view. Miss Nightingale, who had done so much to improve the status of nursing and nurses, argued that nursing was a calling in which character and dedication were more important than factual knowledge, and that these two vital qualities could not be assessed by any form of examination. Paget and his good friend, the physician Sir Henry Acland, both believed that registration of nurses was desirable and inevitable. As office-bearers in two nurses' organisations—the British Nurses' Association and the Royal Jubilee Institute—they had to tread warily in their dealings with Miss Nightingale. In 1893 Paget wrote to Acland:

I think it is only a question whether [registration] is to be granted at once or a few years hence. . . . Many brothers become doctors, or dentists, and are registered: their sisters become nurses, and are not registered. Or in the same family, one sister takes a medical qualification and is registered, another becomes a nurse, and she cannot be registered. The contrast is becoming ridiculous as well as unjust, and must soon come to an end. . . . I should be 'for' registration; but am much more 'against' being induced to attend a meeting about it; the older I grow, the more I dislike speaking.[2]

Four years later the question had still not been settled, although Miss Nightingale was beginning to concede that some form of registration could eventually become necessary. Paget's letter to Acland, who lived in Oxford, shows how weary he had become of the protracted dispute:

I am glad that something has brought me the pleasure of a letter from you—the only pleasure I have to thank [the Royal British Nurses' Association] for. I had the same papers sent to me, and had decided that the best plan for me was to send no answer. Your letter, implying the same wish in your mind, makes me sure that we are both of us right. I have never taken any share in the business of the Association; and have been strictly a Vice-President; and have not studied any of the reasons of the dispute or been near any of the meetings about it. It is too feminine for me, and I have always pleaded that I was trying to do a fair share of such work in the Queen Victoria's Jubilee Institute. I am, thank God, very well—only very old; but this with no pain and with only such signs of warning as I may be very thankful for. I wish you may find some safe and happy reason for coming to London. Then I may see you: for I can hardly hope in winter weather to come to Oxford. Goodbye, dear Acland, God be with you.[3]

Final publications
In 1891 Longmans published Paget's *Study of Old Case-books,* the project that had been one of his major interests for the previous five years. This collection of essays contains his mature re-assessment of observations made during his fifty years in practice. Some of the essays are of lasting interest because they reflect social attitudes of the second half of the nineteenth century. Paget was considered to be rather unorthodox in his belief that girls should be permitted to grow up like boys, enjoying games in the open air. He develops this theme in his essay *On Spines Suspected of Deformity:*

Among the fears of disease for which one is consulted, none is more frequent than that of lateral curvature of the spine. These fears are felt, especially, by mothers among the richer classes; and usually the fear is only for their daughters' spines. It is thought essential to the welfare of a young lady that her spine should be straight, and her form not notably unsymmetrical, and that she would habitually sit upright with her back unsupported. There is no such thought for young gentlemen, and it appears to be, chiefly, a consequence of this difference, that in the well-to-do classes lateral curvature of the spine is at least twenty times more frequent in girls than in boys. For mothers seldom look at their sons' spines; and they let them sit with their elbows on the table, loll back in their chairs, and lie flat on their stomachs, and do many more such prudent things as in the daughters would be deemed shameful. Thus boys' spines grow straight; the muscles helping to support them are not over-tired, or, when they are, they can be rested in any comfortable posture. . . . The folly and the mischief of this contrast are happily becoming known: the good rule of letting girls grow up like boys is becoming more and more widely observed, and a larger proportion of them are well-formed, graceful, and strong. Still, the unfounded fears of deformity of the spine are far too frequent, and they are main-tained, in many instances, by the existence of slight deviations from the supposed pattern-shape which are quite harmless. It seems to be assumed by some that all spines should have curves and other characters exactly similar to those which are seen in artists' models or in anatomical plates. It is much more probable that there are as many varieties of healthy spines as of healthy chins or cheeks, or as many in the human species as in the horse or ox.[4]

Paget's article on Pasteur, in which he reviewed the life's work of that great man, was published in *Nature* on 26 March, 1891. It is an authoritative account of Pasteur's contributions to science and medicine. He tells how Pasteur's study of the process of fermentation provided the basis for Lister's now universally accepted teaching, and of the resultant transformation of surgery:

> It is impossible to estimate the number of the thousands of lives that are thus annually saved by practices which are the direct consequences of Pasteur's observations on the action of living ferments, and of Lister's application of them. In the practice of surgery alone, they are by far the most important of the means by which the risks of death or serious illness after wounds are reduced to less than half of what they were thirty years ago; and of the means by which a large number of operations, such as, at that time, would have been so dangerous that no prudent surgeon would have performed them, are now safely done.[5]

His last published article appeared in the *British Medical Journal* in 1894. It was a report of an address he gave to the Abernethian Society, just sixty years after he read to that Society his paper on *Trichina spiralis*.

Failing health
Declining physical strength caused him to curtail his activities. Lydia Paget's health was also failing. In 1888 Paget received pressing invitations to visit friends in the United States, but his wife was not strong enough to undertake the long sea voyage, and he would not go without her. In the same year the long holidays on the Continent came to an end, when the family visited Switzerland together for the last time. Paget's pleasure in Swiss scenery and wildflowers, and in the good food at the inns, was undiminished, but the walks he took were shorter than the day-long excursions he had enjoyed in earlier years. At the beginning of the holiday the sudden illness of a member of the party had been a sharp reminder to Paget of his reliance on the help of friends in such crises. Although the patient made a rapid recovery, the episode reinforced his decision that future holidays would be spent in England or Wales.

In 1891 he made a last brief working-trip to the Continent. He was called upon at short notice to go to Rome for a consultation. His only sight of that great city gave him little pleasure, as he said in a letter to a member of the family:

I could not have imagined a week ago that I should be writing to you from Rome; yet here I certainly am, thank God, and am well, and yet not enjoying myself; for the unhappiness of being here alone is greater than the happiness of seeing things which, if any of 'mine' had been with me, I should have been more glad than I could have expressed in seeing. I now want more than anything to be at home again.[6]

Nostalgic visits to familiar places now gave him more satisfaction than seeing new sights. In 1888 he had returned to Yarmouth and seen again the family home. The house on the Quay had been acquired by the Corporation of Great Yarmouth for its School of Science and Art, and was greatly changed, as was the town itself:

We all had a long walk through the town this morning, and I had great pleasure in remembering nearly every house we passed, and those who had lived in it; and nearly as much pain in seeing their changes, all drifting down, good houses becoming counting-houses, and handsome frontages built-out in shops, and all the signs of active foreign commerce gone. The change in the town is nearly complete—a busy and important place of commerce and shipbuilding is a fishing-place and seaside watering-place. We went over the old house, and could trace what was beautiful in its forms, and all the arrangements of its rooms: but not one fragment of its decorations remains except a beautiful Italian marble chimney-piece, and the drawers and closets of the great store-room.[7]

Stephen Paget said of his father that London never quite effaced Yarmouth in him. 'He had an eye for a ship; and kept, all his life, his knowledge of shipping, his love of the sea, and a trace of Norfolk accent.'[8]

In 1891 James persuaded George to join him in another visit to Yarmouth. These two were now the only surviving members of Samuel Paget's immediate family; Frederick, the wanderer, had died in 1867, Patty in 1881, and Kate in 1885. As George and James strolled through the scenes of their childhood they recalled the sad and the happy events of the distant past, each brother filling in the gaps in the other's memory. Three months later George dined at Harewood Place on the occasion of James's seventy-eighth birthday. A few days later George fell ill with pneumonia and on 29 January, 1892, he died. In a letter to an old friend James wrote a tribute to this brother who, of all his brothers and sisters, had been the closest to him:

He was, indeed, admirable in all his life, and those most near to him might well think him faultless. He was, for many years, the main stay of the whole family; the only one who had power to help the rest. But for him, I doubt whether I could have studied my profession, and yet, in all the years that have since passed, I have never heard a word or seen a look that could remind me of my deep obligation to him. His end was like his whole life—gentle, pious, watchful for the happiness of all around him—just such as one may wish to imitate with truth.[9]

Now that all of James's children except the youngest, Mary, had married and left the family home, the house in Harewood Place had become too large. Many of Paget's contemporaries had retired to the country but, much as he enjoyed country holidays, Paget remained a lover of cities, and particularly of London. In 1893 James, Lydia, and Mary left Harewood Place and moved to a smaller house at 5, Park Square West, Regent's Park. It satisfied Lydia's requirement of 'a little cottage with a big garden'. On 23 May of the following year James and Lydia celebrated their golden wedding. He left no account of the celebrations, but there remains a letter, written by Lydia on the occasion of the forty-fourth anniversary of their engagement, that tells of their unfailing love for each other:

Forty-four years since we were engaged! and forty-four years it seems, I must own, with its crowd of untold blessings, the times of sore trial, the poverty, the riches (comparatively), the times of weariness, the elation of feeling rested, the onward progress of our most dear children, the many loved ones gone, the far greater number spared to our exceeding joy, the many changes that have marked our lives. And what a strange thing, in this imperfect state of being, to be able to speak of one's having more gentle love, more confidence, more sweet dependence on one, than ever. The long years have not worn all these great sources of joy out, but the stream of even, mutual love seems uninterrupted.[10]

On 7 January, 1895, Lydia Paget died, 'as gently and simply as she had lived'. Her loss accelerated the ageing process in her husband. James now neither desired nor dreaded death, but resigned himself to the will of God. Although the religion his parents taught their children was that of simple piety, in later life he became quite a student of theology, and in his last years, when he lost his inclination for other reading, he kept close at hand his New Testament and several of his favourite theological works. In November 1897 he wrote to his old friend, Sir Henry Acland:

I wish I could hope to see you soon: but I fear this cannot be in

Oxford. My infirmities increase so rapidly that I cannot hope to travel so far, in weather so nearly cold as we must have in winter. They increase, thank God, without pain, but not without evidence or warning. And I try to use their warnings rightly, using especially what you gave me last year—Dr Pusey's book of prayers edited by Dr Liddon, and good Bishop Andrewes' Meditations. I could have, I think, no better human guidance. May

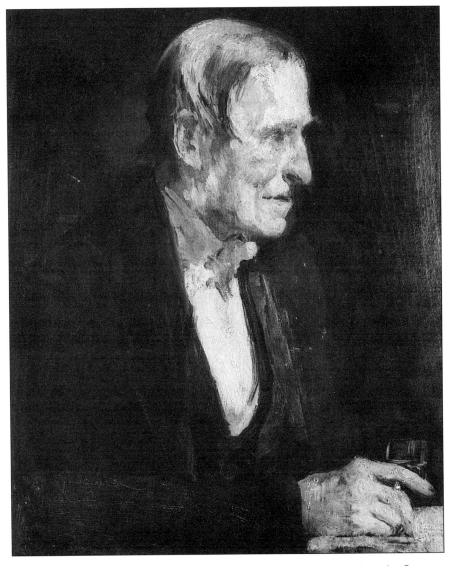

Sir James Paget, 1894. By SJ Solomon, study for the larger painting An Octave for Mr Ernest Hart. *(Wellcome Institute).*

God bless them and guide me to their just use—adding this to His many mercies.[11]

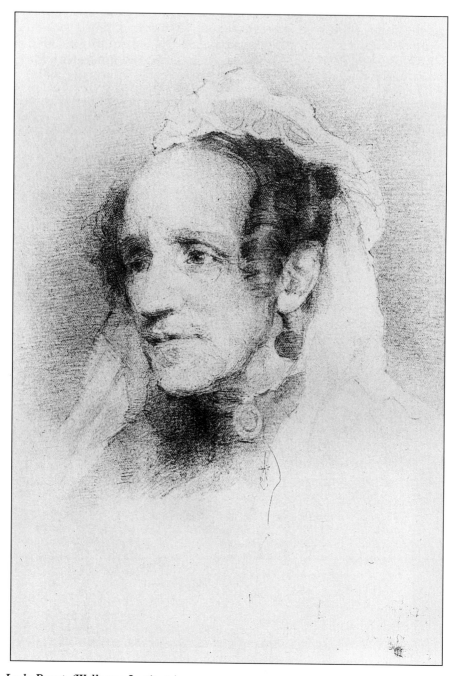

Lady Paget. (Wellcome Institute).

This was the last letter he ever wrote. Soon afterwards he became so weak that he could not write, and even speech was difficult, although his mind remained as lucid as ever. Sir James Paget died on 30 December, 1899. His funeral service in Westminster Abbey was attended by distinguished men and women who had known him when his career was at its zenith. Outside the Abbey medical students formed a guard of honour for a man they had never seen, but whose life was an inspiration to their profession.

References

Chapter 1
The House on the Quay

1 Alfred Paget. *The Pagets of Great Yarmouth—A Family Chronicle.* (Unpublished) p1.
2 Ibid. p5.
3 Stephen Paget. *Memoirs and Letters of Sir James Paget.* (3rd Edn)
London: Longmans, Green & Co, 1903. p5.
4 Ibid. p2.
5 Alfred Paget. *The Pagets of Great Yarmouth—A Family Chronicle*
(Unpublished) p31.
6 Ibid. p32.
7 Ibid. p33.
8 Stephen Paget. *Memoirs and Letters of Sir James Paget.* (3rd Edn)
London: Longmans, Green & Co, 1903. p4.
9 Ibid. pp6–9.
10 Ibid. p9.
11 Ibid. p17.
12 Alfred Paget. *The Pagets of Great Yarmouth—A Family Chronicle.* (Unpublished) p8.
13 Ibid. p35.
14 Stephen Paget. *Memoirs and Letters of Sir James Paget.* (3rd Edn) London: Longmans, Green & Co, 1903. p10.

Chapter 2
The Apprentice Surgeon-Apothecary

1 Stephen Paget. *Memoirs and Letters of Sir James Paget.* (3rd Edn). London: Longmans, Green & Co, 1903. p20.
2 Ibid. p21.
3 Ibid. p23.
4 Ibid. p22.
5 Ibid. p23.
6 Ibid. p24.
7 Ibid. p24.
8 Alfred Paget. *The Pagets of Great Yarmouth—A Family Chronicle.* (Unpublished) p43.
9 Ibid. p44.
10 Ibid. p53.

11 Stephen Paget. *Memoirs and Letters of Sir James Paget.* (3rd Edn) London: Longmans, Green & Co, 1903. p25.

12 Ibid. p26.

13 Ibid. p28.

14 Alfred Paget. *The Pagets of Great Yarmouth—A Family Chronicle.* (Unpublished) p61.

15 Stephen Paget. *Memoirs and Letters of Sir James Paget.* (3rd Edn) London: Longmans, Green & Co, 1903. pp 19, 20, 29–30.

Chapter 3
The Student in London

1 James Paget. *St Bartholomew's Hospital and School Fifty Years Ago.* London: The Medical Magazine Association, 1905. p6.

2 Stephen Paget. *Memoirs and Letters* of *Sir James Paget.* (3rd Edn) London: Longmans, Green & Co, 1903. pp45–47.

3 James Paget. *St Bartholomew's Hospital and School Fifty Years Ago.* London: The Medical Magazine Association, 1905. p29.

4 Stephen Paget. *Memoirs and Letters of Sir James Paget.* (3rd Edn) London: Longmans, Green & Co, 1903. p42.

5 Ibid. p43.

6 Ibid. p55.

7 James Paget to Charles Paget, 11 Feb. 1835. Collected Papers of Sir James Paget, held at the Royal College of Surgeons, London.

8 Stephen Paget. *Memoirs and Letters of Sir James Paget.* (3rd Edn) London: Longmans, Green & Co, 1903. p56.

9 Ibid. p54.

10 *Report of Commissioners for City of London Inquiring Concerning Charities,* 1837. p56.

11 Ibid. p58.

12 James Paget. *St Bartholomew's Hospital and School Fifty Years Ago.* London: The Medical Magazine Association, 1905. p7.

13 Ibid. p26.

14 Ibid. p18.

15 Ibid. p17.

16 Ibid. p23.

17 Stephen Paget. *Memoirs and Letters of Sir James Paget.* (3rd Edn) London: Longmans, Green & Co, 1903. p61.

18 Ibid. p67.

Chapter 4
Working, Waiting, and Hoping

1 Stephen Paget. *Memoirs and Letters of Sir James Paget.* (3rd Edn) London: Longmans, Green & Co, 1903. p69.
2 Samuel Paget to Revd Henry North, 24 Oct. 1836. Paget Family Papers, Wellcome Foundation, London.
3 Stephen Paget. *Memoirs and Letters of Sir James Paget.* (3rd Edn) London: Longmans, Green & Co, 1903. p94.
4 Ibid. p97.
5 Ibid. pp 98–101.
6 Ibid. p101.
7 Ibid. p77.
8 Ibid. p73.
9 Ibid. p75.
10 Ibid. p105.
11 Ibid. p79.
12 Ibid. p104.
13 Ibid. p106.
14 Ibid. p106.
15 Sir James Clark and Sir Charles Clarke. *Lancet;* 37: 19 October 1839.
16 Stephen Paget. *Memoirs and Letters of Sir James Paget.* (3rd Edn) London: Longmans, Green & Co, 1903. p80.
17 Ibid. p111.
18 Alfred Paget.*The Pagets of Great Yarmouth—A Family Chronicle.* (Unpublished) p74.
19 Ibid. p76.
20 Stephen Paget. *Memoirs and Letters of Sir James Paget.* (3rd Edn) London: Longmans, Green & Co, 1903. p113.
21 Ibid. p85.
22 *The Times.* 3 February 1842.
23 Stephen Paget. *Memoirs and Letters of Sir James Paget.* (3rd Edn) London: Longmans, Green & Co, 1903. p117.

Chapter 5
The College Warden

1 Stephen Paget. *Memoirs and Letters of Sir James Paget.* (3rd Edn) London: Longmans, Green & Co, 1903. p122.
2 Ibid. p123.
3 Ibid. p149.
4 Ibid. p150.
5 Ibid. p146.

6 Alfred Paget. *The Pagets of Great Yarmouth—A Family Chronicle.* (Unpublished) p94.
7 Stephen Paget. *Memoirs and Letters of Sir James Paget.* (3rd Edn) London: Longmans, Green & Co, 1903. p128.
8 James Paget. *Records of Harvey, in Extracts from the Journals of the Royal Hospital of St Bartholomew.* London: John Churchill, 1846. p13.
9 Ibid. p41.
10 Ibid. p42.
11 Stephen Paget. *Memoirs and Letters of Sir James Paget.* (3rd Edn) London: Longmans, Green & Co, 1903. p157.
12 Ibid. p176.
13 Ibid. p155.
14 Alfred Paget.*The Pagets of Great Yarmouth—A Family Chronicle.* (Unpublished) pp115, 116–117.
15 Ibid. p112.
16 Ibid. p122.
17 Pathological Catalogue of the Museum of the Royal College of Surgeons. 1849.
18 Stephen Paget. *Memoirs and Letters of Sir James Paget.* (3rd Edn) London: Longmans, Green & Co, 1903. p165.
19 Howard Marsh and Oliver Pemberton. In Memoriam: Sir William Savory. *St Bartholomew's Hospital Reports.* 1895, **xxxi.**
20 Janet Nye. Elizabeth Blackwell. *St Bartholomew's Hospital Journal.* April, 1953.
21 Ibid.
22 James Paget. What Becomes of Medical Students. *St Bartholomew's Hospital Reports,* 1871; **vii**; 67.
23 James Paget. On the Recent Progress of Anatomy and its Influence on Surgery. *Medical Times and Gazette, New Series,* 12 July 1851; **No 54**.
24 Ibid.
25 Stephen Paget. *Memoirs and Letters of Sir James Paget.* (3rd Edn) London: Longmans, Green & Co, 1903. p128–130.

Chapter 6
A Liberal Measure of Success

1 Stephen Paget. *Memoirs and Letters of Sir James Paget.* (3rd Edn) London: Longmans, Green & Co, 1903. p206.
2 Ibid. p212.
3 Ibid. p208.
4 Ibid. p215.
5 Ibid. p218.

6 Ibid. p218.
7 BW Richardson MD and Wade Hampton Frost MD. *Snow on Cholera, A Reprint of two Papers by John Snow MD, Together With a Biological Memoir and an Introduction.* New York, London: Hafner Publishing Co, 1965. p74.
8 Sir Edward Cook. *The Life of Florence Nightingale.* London: Macmillan, 1913. p434.
9 Stephen Paget. *Memoirs and Letters of Sir James Paget.* (3rd Edn) London: Longmans, Green & Co, 1903. p183.
10 Ibid. p232.
11 James Paget. What Becomes of Medical Students. *St Bartholomew's Hospital Reports,* 1871; **vii**: p67.
12 Ibid.
13 Stephen Paget. *Memoirs and Letters of Sir James Paget.* (3rd Edn) London: Longmans, Green & Co, 1903. p228.
14 Ibid. p220.
15 Ibid. p259.
16 Ibid. p258.
17 Ibid. p236.
18 Ibid. p237.
19 Ibid. p255.
20 James Paget. Dissection Poisons. *Lancet,* 10 June 1871. p775.
21 Ibid.

Chapter 7
Recognition and Rewards

1 Stephen Paget. *Memoirs and Letters of Sir James Paget.* (3rd Edn) London: Longmans, Green & Co, 1903. p251.
2 GWE Russell. *Portraits of the Seventies.* London: T Fisher Unwin, 1916.
3 Stephen Paget. *Memoirs and Letters of Sir James Paget.* (3rd Edn) London: Longmans, Green & Co, 1903. p261.
4 Ibid. p252.
5 James Paget. On Disease of the Mammary Areola Preceding Cancer of the Mammary Gland. *St Bartholomew's Hospital Reports,* 1874; **vol x**: p87.
6 James Paget. On a Form of Chronic Inflammation of the Bones (Osteitis Deformans). *Medico-Chirurgical Transactions,* 1876; **vol ix**: p37.
7 James Paget. On the Recent Progress of Anatomy and its Influence on Surgery. *Medical Times and Gazette, New Series,* 12 July 1851; **No 54.**
8 Henry Butlin. On the Minute Anatomy of Two Breasts. *Medico-chirurgical Transactions,* 1876, p107.

9 Stephen Paget. *Memoirs and Letters of Sir James Paget.* (3rd Edn) London: Longmans, Green & Co, 1903. p413.
10 Ibid. p407.
11 Ibid. p409.
12 Sir Rickman Godlee. *Lord Lister.* (2nd Edn) Oxford University Press, 1924. p378.
13 Ibid. p379.
14 Calendar of the Royal College of Surgeons of England. 1940.
15 Peter W Verco. *Masons, Millers, and Medicine.* Adelaide: Lutheran Publishing House, 1976. p86.
16 James Paget. *The Hunterian Oration of 1877.* London: Longmans, Green and Co, 1877. p5.
17 Ibid. p20.
18 Ibid. p26.
19 Ibid. p34.
20 *The Times.* 1 Jan 1900.
21 Stephen Paget. *Memoirs and Letters of Sir James Paget.* (3rd Edn) London: Longmans, Green & Co, 1903. p235.
22 Sir Rickman Godlee. *Lord Lister.* (2nd Edn) Oxford University Press, 1924. p446.
23 Stephen Paget. *Memoirs and Letters of Sir James Paget.* (3rd Edn) London: Longmans, Green & Co, 1903. p317.
24 Ibid. p321.
25 Ibid. p324.

Chapter 8
The Committee Man

1 James Paget. The Vivisection Question. In: *Selected Essays and Addresses.* London: Longmans, Green and Co, 1902.
2 Stephen Paget. *Memoirs and Letters of Sir James Paget.* (3rd Edn) London: Longmans, Green & Co, 1903. p400.
3 Ibid. p349.
4 Ibid. p354.
5 Ibid. p355.
6 Stephen Paget. *Sir Victor Horsley.* London: Constable, 1919.
7 Stephen Paget. *Memoirs and Letters of Sir James Paget.* (3rd Edn) London: Longmans, Green & Co, 1903. p384.
8 Arthur Wollaston Hutton. *The Vaccination Question.* London: Methuen, 1895.
9 Stephen Paget. *Memoirs and Letters of Sir James Paget.* (3rd Edn) London: Longmans, Green & Co, 1903. p385.
10 Ibid. p335.
11 Alfred Franklin. A Bart's Woman: 1865. *St Bartholomew's Hospital Journal,* 1 November 1931.

12 Stephen Paget. *Memoirs and Letters of Sir James Paget.* (3rd Edn) London: Longmans, Green & Co, 1903. p298.

13 Henry Scott Holland. *Personal Studies.* London: Wells, Gardner, Darton and Co Ltd, 1905. p198.

14 Charles Newman. *The Evolution of Medical Education in the Nineteenth   Century.* Oxford University Press, 1957. p82.

Chapter 9
The Work is Finished

1 Stephen Paget. *Memoirs and Letters of Sir James Paget.* (3rd Edn) London: Longmans, Green & Co, 1903. p202.

2 Ibid. p401.

3 Ibid. p425.

4 James Paget. *Studies of Old Case-books.* London: Longmans, 1891.

5 James Paget. Louis Pasteur. *Nature,* 26 March 1891: **No 1117, vol 43:** p481

6 Stephen Paget. *Memoirs and Letters of Sir James Paget.* (3rd Edn) London: Longmans, Green & Co, 1903. p392.

7 Ibid. p379.

8 Ibid. p38.

9 Ibid. p399.

10 Ibid. p403.

11 Ibid. p425.

Bibliography

Contemporary Sources

A. Family Papers
1. Articles and letters by Sir James Paget, in the possession of the Royal College of Surgeons of England, Lincoln's Inn Fields, London.
2. Paget Family Papers, in the possession of the Wellcome Institute for the History of Medicine, Euston Road, London.
3. Paget, Alfred. *The Pagets of Great Yarmouth—A Family Chronicle.* (unpublished). A copy is held at the Norwich Library.

B. Official Documents
1. Report of Commissioners for the City of London Inquiring Concerning Charities, 1837.
2. Report of a Committee appointed by the Local Government Board to inquire into M. Pasteur's treatment of Hydrophobia 1887 (c. 5087) LXVI, 429.
3. Royal Commission appointed to inquire into the subject of Vaccination. Final Report 1896 (c. 8270) XLVII, 889

C. Newspapers, Medical and Scientific Journals
The British Medical Journal
Lancet
Medical Times and Gazette
Medico-Chirurgical Transactions
Nature
Nineteenth Century
St Bartholomew's Hospital Journal
St Bartholomew's Hospital Reports
The Times

D. Books
Bettany GT. *Eminent Doctors, Their Lives and Their Work.* London: John Hogg, 1886.
Butcher Richard G. *Essays and Reports on Surgery.* Dublin: Fannin and Co, 1865.
Cooper Sir Astley. *The Principles and Practice of Surgery.* London: 1837.
Cullen William. *First Lines of the Practice of Physic.* (Edited by James Crawford Gregory). Edinburgh: 1829.
Edwards Edward J. *Small-pox and Vaccination in Europe.* London: HK Lewis, 1902.

Hutton, Arthur Wollaston. *The Vaccination Question.*
London: Methuen, 1895.

Paget Charles E. *Some Lectures by the Late Sir George Paget.*
Cambridge: Macmillan and Bowes, 1893.

Paget James. *The Hunterian Oration of 1877.* London:
Longmans, Green and Co, 1877.

Paget James. *Records of Harvey, in Extracts from the
Journals of the Royal Hospital of St Bartholomew.* London:
John Churchill, 1846.

Paget James. *Studies of Old Case-books.* London: Longmans,
Green and Co, 1891.

Paget Stephen. *The Memoirs and Letters of Sir James Paget.*
(3rd Edn) London: Longmans, Green and Co, 1903.

Paget Stephen. *John Hunter.* London: Fisher, Unwin, 1903.

Palmer, Charles John. *Perlustrations of Great Yarmouth,
with Gorleston and Southtown.* Great Yarmouth: 1872.

Later Books and Articles

Bishop WJ. *The Evolution of the General Practitioner in
England.* Science, Medicine, and History, edited by E A
Underwood. London: Oxford University Press, 1953.

Brockington C Fraser. *A Short History of Public Health.*
London: J and A Churchill, 1956.

Cook Sir Edward. *The Life of Florence Nightingale.* London:
Macmillan, 1913.

Cope Sir Zachary. *Florence Nightingale and the Doctors.*
London: Spottiswood Ballantyne and Co Ltd, 1938.

Cope Sir Zachary. *The Royal College of Surgeons of
England—A History.* London: Anthony Blond, 1959.

Cope Sir Zachary. *A History of the Acute Abdomen.* London:
Oxford University Press, 1965.

Denny Sir Lionel. *The Royal Hospitals of the City of London.*
Annals of the Royal College of Surgeons of England, Vol 52,
1973.

Foster Janet. *Bart's in Paget's Day.* (Unpublished) Archives
of St Bartholomew's Hospital.

Franklin A White. A Bart's Woman, 1865. *St Bartholomew's
Hospital Journal,* 39, 1931–2

Frazer WM. *History of English Public Health.* London:
Tindall and Cox, 1950.

French Richard D. *Vivisection and Medical Science in
Victorian Society.* Princeton University Press, 1975.

Godlee Sir Rickman John. *Lord Lister.* London: Oxford
University Press, 1924.

Greene, Nicholas M. *Anaesthesia and the Development of*

Surgery (1846–1896). Anaesthesia and Analgesia, 1979; **58**, i.

Grey Turner George. *The Paget Tradition. New England Journal of Medicine,* 24 September 1931.

Guthrie Douglas. *Lord Lister.* Edinburgh: Livingstone, 1949.

Haight, Gordon S. *George Eliot—A Biography.* London: Oxford University Press, 1968.

Harding Rains AJ. *Editorial Comment in Annals of the Royal College of Surgeons of England,* January, 1982; **Vol 64, No 1**

Holland Henry Scott. *Personal Studies.* London: Wells, Gardner, Darton and Co, 1905.

Kerling Nellie J. *St Bartholomew's and Epidemics in the City of London. St Bartholomew's Hospital Journal,* 1971: **75**.

Mc Innes EM. *St Thomas's Hospital.* London: George Allen and Unwin, 1963.

McKay WJS. *Lawson Tait: His Life and Work.* London: 1922.

Manton Jo. *Elizabeth Garret Anderson.* London: Methuen, 1965.

Medvei Victor Cornelius and Thornton John L. (eds) *The Royal Hospital of St Bartholomew.* London: 1974.

Newman Charles. *The Evolution of Medical Education in the Nineteenth Century.* London: Oxford University Press, 1957.

Nye Janet.*Elizabeth Blackwell. St Bartholomew's Hospital Journal,* 1953; **57.**

Paget Stephen. *Sir Victor Horsley.* London: Constable, 1919.

Parish HJ. *A History of Immunisation.* Edinburgh and London: E and S Livingstone, 1965.

Peterson M Jeanne. *The Medical Profession in Mid-Victorian London.* University of California Press, 1978.

Richardson BW and Frost Wade Hampton. *Snow on Cholera, Being a Reprint of Two Papers by John Snow MD, Together With a Biographical Memoir and an Introduction.* New York and London: Hafner Publishing Co, 1965.

Risley Mary. *The House of Healing.* London: Robert Hale Ltd, 1961.

Russell GWE. *Portraits of the Seventies.* London: Fisher Unwin Ltd, 1916.

Shepherd John A. *Spencer Wells—The Life and Work of a Victorian Surgeon.* London: E and S Livingstone, 1965.

Shepherd JA. *Lawson Tait: The Rebellious Surgeon.* Lawrence, Kansas: Coronado Press, 1980.

Smith Harold. *The Society for the Diffusion of Useful Knowledge, 1826–1846.* Halifax, Nova Scotia: 1974.

Truax Rhoda. *Joseph Lister, Father of Modern Surgery.* London: George and Harrap, 1947.

Verco Peter W. *Masons, Millers, and Medicine.* Adelaide: Lutheran Press, 1976.

Index